Coping with Thyr

Mark Greener spent a decade in biomedic
Magazine for GPs in 1989. Since then he has written on health and biology
for magazines worldwide for patients, healthcare professionals and sci-
entists. He is the author of 15 other books, including *The Heart Attack
Survival Guide* (2012) and *The Holistic Health Handbook* (2013), both for
Sheldon Press. Mark lives with his wife, three children and two cats in a
Cambridgeshire village.

Overcoming Common Problems Series

Selected titles

A full list of titles is available from Sheldon Press,
36 Causton Street, London SW1P 4ST and on our website at
www.sheldonpress.co.uk

Breast Cancer: Your treatment choices
Dr Terry Priestman

Chronic Fatigue Syndrome: What you need to know
Dr Megan A. Arroll

Cider Vinegar
Margaret Hills

Coping Successfully with Chronic Illness: Your healing plan
Neville Shone

Coping Successfully with Shyness
Margaret Oakes, Professor Robert Bor and Dr Carina Eriksen

Coping with Difficult Families
Dr Jane McGregor and Tim McGregor

Coping with Epilepsy
Dr Pamela Crawford and Fiona Marshall

Coping with Guilt
Dr Windy Dryden

Coping with Liver Disease
Mark Greener

Coping with Memory Problems
Dr Sallie Baxendale

Coping with Obsessive Compulsive Disorder
Professor Kevin Gournay, Rachel Piper and Professor Paul Rogers

Coping with Schizophrenia
Professor Kevin Gournay and Debbie Robson

Coping with Thyroid Disease
Mark Greener

Depressive Illness – the Curse of the Strong
Dr Tim Cantopher

The Diabetes Healing Diet
Mark Greener and Christine Craggs-Hinton

The Empathy Trap: Understanding Antisocial Personalities
Dr Jane McGregor and Tim McGregor

Epilepsy: Complementary and alternative treatments
Dr Sallie Baxendale

Fibromyalgia: Your Treatment Guide
Christine Craggs-Hinton

Hay Fever: How to beat it
Dr Paul Carson

The Heart Attack Survival Guide
Mark Greener

Helping Elderly Relatives
Jill Eckersley

The Holistic Health Handbook
Mark Greener

How to Eat Well When You Have Cancer
Jane Freeman

How to Stop Worrying
Dr Frank Tallis

The Irritable Bowel Diet Book
Rosemary Nicol

Living with Complicated Grief
Professor Craig A. White

Living with IBS
Nuno Ferreira and David T. Gillanders

Making Sense of Trauma: How to tell your story
Dr Nigel C. Hunt and Dr Sue McHale

Overcoming Fear: With mindfulness
Deborah Ward

Overcoming Loneliness
Alice Muir

Overcoming Stress
Professor Robert Bor, Dr Carina Eriksen and Dr Sara Chaudry

Overcoming Worry and Anxiety
Dr Jerry Kennard

Physical Intelligence: How to take charge of your weight
Dr Tom Smith

The Self-Esteem Journal
Alison Waines

Ten Steps to Positive Living
Dr Windy Dryden

Transforming Eight Deadly Emotions into Healthy Ones
Dr Windy Dryden

Treating Arthritis: The drug-free way
Margaret Hills and Christine Horner

Treating Arthritis: The supplements guide
Julia Davies

Understanding Yourself and Others: Practical ideas from the world of coaching
Bob Thomson

When Someone You Love Has Depression: A handbook for family and friends
Barbara Baker

Overcoming Common Problems

Coping with Thyroid Disease

MARK GREENER

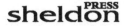

First published in Great Britain in 2014

Sheldon Press .
36 Causton Street
London SW1P 4ST
www.sheldonpress.co.uk

British Library Cataloguing-in-Publication Data
A catalogue record for this book is available from the British Library

ISBN 978-1-84709-294-6
eBook ISBN 978-1-84709-295-3

Typeset by Fakenham Prepress Solutions, Fakenham, Norfolk NR21 8NN
First printed in Great Britain by Ashford Colour Press
Subsequently digitally reprinted in Great Britain

eBook by Fakenham Prepress Solutions, Fakenham, Norfolk NR21 8NN

Produced on paper from sustainable forests

As always, to Rose, Rory, Ophelia and Yasmin

Contents

Note to the reader

This is not a medical book and is not intended to replace advice from your doctor. Consult your pharmacist or doctor if you believe you have any of the symptoms described, and if you think you might need medical help.

Introduction

Goitres – swellings, sometimes massive, of the butterfly-shaped thyroid gland, which lies in front of the trachea (windpipe) just below your Adam's apple – are one of the most recognizable diseases, even if you are not a doctor or nurse. Indeed, Chinese physicians described goitres as long ago as 2700 BC.[1] Later, Roman armies crossing the Alps reported that in some villages almost everyone had a goitre.[2] Later explorers, missionaries and doctors reported goitres in people living in Africa, Asia and South America.[3] Closer to home, goitres were so widespread in the Pennines, they became known as 'Derbyshire neck'.[4]

Today, thyroid diseases remain common: more than 1 in 10 women develop thyroid disease at some point, for example.[5] About 1.6 million people in the UK take chronic (long-term) levothyroxine to replace missing thyroid hormone;[5] that's more people than the populations of Birmingham and Liverpool together. Furthermore, some thyroid diseases seem to be becoming even more common. For example, Cancer Research says that the number of thyroid cancers among women quadrupled during the last 40 years. In 2010, doctors diagnosed about one person every 3 hours with thyroid cancer.

However, unless you develop goitre, the signs of thyroid disease are often subtle, insidious and ambiguous. As a result, doctors can easily misdiagnose thyroid disease. Some people suffer for years from distressing symptoms – including fatigue, insomnia, depression, dry skin, thinning hair and weight gain – caused by undetected and untreated thyroid problems. Doctors may also misdiagnose thyroid disease as the 'baby blues', period problems or chronic fatigue. In some cases, the treatments offered (such as antidepressants) 'paper over the cracks' without really tackling the cause. And nobody really knows how many people live with thyroid symptoms but never seek professional help.

Indeed, increasingly sensitive tests reveal a growing number of people with 'subclinical' thyroid disease. It sounds almost banal. Yet subclinical thyroid disease might increase your risk of potentially fatal heart disease. This book aims to help you get the care you need. Once a doctor diagnoses your thyroid disease, the book offers some suggestions to help you live a full and fulfilled life.

Meet your thyroid

The thyroid gland controls how hard other parts of your body work by producing hormones (chemical messengers) that increase the energy burnt off by almost every tissue and organ.[6] Hormones produced by the thyroid ensure that your heart pumps properly, that you can breathe and move, and that your liver and kidneys get rid of toxic waste. Thyroid hormones are essential for reproduction and to make sure your baby is healthy. Thyroid hormones help keep you looking well and attractive – low levels can leave you with dry, brittle and thin hair, and dry, coarse and puffy skin. Thyroid hormones even ensure your weight remains stable. Tight rings and clothes can be one of the first signs that your thyroid is not working properly.

In other words, a healthy thyroid is essential for your well-being. Langer and Scheer recount that Victorian doctors in Harley Street gave their 'elderly and failing patients' a boost by feeding them sandwiches containing raw thyroid glands from animals (see 'Further reading').

So how does this link to goitres? Our bodies need a range of minerals. Iron in haemoglobin carries oxygen around our bodies. Our nerves and muscles need potassium and sodium to work properly. Some enzymes – specialized proteins that ensure that the millions of chemical reactions that keep us alive work properly – need tiny amounts of more exotic minerals. Manganese, for example, is involved in the production of thyroxine, one thyroid hormone, and zinc boosts the immune system and helps repair damaged tissue.[7]

In 1811, the French chemist Bernard Courtois discovered another essential mineral – iodine.[3] The name comes from the Greek word for violet or purple, the colour of iodine vapour. Goitre can indicate that you are not getting enough iodine, which is essential for the production of thyroid hormone.

From about 1600 BC, Chinese healers treated goitres with burnt sponge and seaweed.[3] Both are rich in iodine, which is why these traditional treatments worked. Indeed, the sea contains most of the world's iodine. Water evaporates from the sea, carrying iodine along with it, and rainfall passes the iodine to the soil. Most of us obtain the iodine our thyroid needs from cereals and milk. However, mountains can be a long way from the sea, and snow and ice leach iodine from the soil. As a result, melt water and food grown on mountains are often low in this essential mineral. That's why goitre is common in many mountainous areas.[3]

Doctors started using iodine supplements to treat goitres in Europe's mountainous regions in the late nineteenth century. During the twentieth century, governments started adding iodine to salt in areas where more than 1 in 20 schoolchildren had enlarged thyroids.[2] Tragically, however, around a third of the world's population – some 2 billion people – still do not get enough iodine, including some of those living in mountainous regions of South East Asia, Latin America and Central Africa.[8,9] Despite our detailed understanding of the thyroid's importance, these people remain at risk of serious and usually preventable health problems.

Even in the UK some of us do not get enough iodine. One recent paper noted that unlike almost every other developed country, no national surveys have monitored iodine status in the UK since the 1940s.[10] Despite this lack of evidence, many doctors believe that people in the UK receive enough iodine in their diet. New research now challenges this complacency. For example, two-thirds of women in the UK seem to be iodine deficient during pregnancy.[10] Tragically, even mild iodine deficiency can leave a baby with a low IQ or can undermine school performance.[10,11] This may imply that many other people may also be deficient in this essential nutrient, although we need a new national survey to be sure. However, not every thyroid disease arises from too little iodine.

Biological civil war

Potentially hazardous bacteria, viruses, fungi and parasites are all around us – in staggering numbers. In her wonderful book *Gulp*, Mary Roach comments that your gut contains about one hundred trillion bacteria – that's about 300 times more than the number of stars in the Milky Way. We usually live in harmony with our bacterial lodgers. The bacteria get somewhere to live and a steady supply of food. In return, they boost the energy released from our diets by about 10 per cent by breaking down foods that we cannot digest.[12] They also help make vitamin K (essential for normal blood clotting),[13] shape our immune responses, prevent our guts from being colonized with other more dangerous bacteria[12] and even help us keep trim[14] and avoid some cancers.[15]

However, not all bacteria are benign, and our immune system protects us from potentially dangerous microorganisms. Occasionally, however, the immune system mistakenly 'turns against' the body. Some so-called 'autoimmune attacks' destroy the thyroid gland, which can cause debilitating symptoms as hormone levels fall. In other cases, the autoimmune attack overstimulates the gland or attacks tissues surrounding the eyes. The resulting increase in hormone levels and eye damage produce the bulging, staring eyes common among people with Graves' disease, one of the most distressing and disfiguring symptoms of thyroid disease.

Furthermore, thyroid diseases are most common among older people: the gland, like many other organs, wears out as we get older. Nevertheless, doctors and patients can easily overlook thyroid disease, partly because the signs and symptoms in older people often mimic common age-related changes and some non-thyroid diseases. For example, hyperthyroidism can cause weight loss – but so can normal ageing, poor nutrition and cancer. Depression may result from grief or hypothyroidism. Memory loss and other cognitive changes may arise from low thyroid hormone levels, age-related memory loss or dementia.[16] Yet an accurate diagnosis is essential to ensure that you receive the most appropriate treatment.

The aim of this book

This book looks at the signs, symptoms, causes and treatment of thyroid disease. We will focus on adults, but mention some of the issues facing children. Many thyroid problems run in families. So if you have a close relative with thyroid disease, try to be especially alert for symptoms in yourself and get these checked by your doctor. Likewise, if you or a close relative have a thyroid disease, you might want to ask a doctor to test your children.

Although thyroid diseases are common, ailments affecting this critical gland attract far less attention than, for example, breast cancer, heart disease or arthritis. As a result, there are numerous controversies in the management of thyroid disease, including who to treat, when and how. And I hope the book will inspire questions. Your nurse, doctor and pharmacist can help guide you through this minefield and answer any queries. You can also talk to patient groups: you can find their contact details in 'Useful addresses'.

As thyroid hormones control how hard every organ and tissue in your body works, you will need to take a holistic approach. Thyroid disease's effects often vary markedly from person to person (one reason why diagnosis can prove so tricky), as well as over time. We will consider the benefits, risks and roles of conventional treatments. We will look at foods that can help your thyroid and at lifestyle and complementary treatments to help you cope with, for example, stress and fatigue. By combining conventional treatments, lifestyle changes and complementary medicines, most people with thyroid disease can live relatively normal, full and fulfilled lives.

A word to the wise

This book does not replace advice from your doctor, nurse or pharmacist, who will offer suggestions, support and treatment tailored to your circumstances. Always see a doctor or nurse if you feel unwell, think that your thyroid disease is getting worse or you worry that you have symptoms that could arise from thyroid disease.

While I have included numerous references from medical and scientific studies, it has been impossible to cite all those I referred to while writing the book. (Apologies to anyone whose work I have missed.) However, throughout the book I have highlighted certain articles to illustrate key points and themes. Some of these may seem rather erudite if you do not have a medical or biological background. However, do not be put off: they are usually understandable if you do some background reading and ask questions.

You can find a summary of the articles by entering the details here: <www.ncbi.nlm.nih.gov/pubmed>. Some full papers are available free online, while some publishers offer cheap access for patients. Larger libraries might stock or allow you to access some better-known medical journals. The better informed you are, the better you will be able to tackle the problems posed by living with thyroid disease.

1

The healthy thyroid

Essentially, your thyroid gland determines how much energy each of the 10 trillion cells in your body uses. Obviously, you need less energy when you are reading or watching television than when you are working out, running for the bus or dealing with a busy, stressful day. In response, the gland tightly controls thyroid hormone production to meet your body's demands. Too little thyroid hormone when you are active and you will not have the energy you need. Too much when you are taking things easy and you may start twitching, feeling nervous or be unable to sit still.

The thyroid's development

The thyroid is the first gland that appears as a baby develops in the womb, beginning to emerge just 22 days or so after conception. The gland starts taking up iodine after 10–11 weeks and begins producing thyroid hormone a couple of weeks later.[17,18] Until this point, the baby depends on thyroid hormone from the mother to ensure its healthy growth and development.[18] Moreover, throughout pregnancy, the developing baby obtains iodine from the mother. That's why it is so important that mothers-to-be and those planning to have a baby receive enough iodine, an issue we will return to in Chapter 8.

The thyroid gland has two lobes, one on each side of the trachea, just below the Adam's apple (Figure 1.1 overleaf). In adults, a normal, healthy thyroid weighs about 20 g. Each lobe is between 4 and 7 cm long, 2.5 cm wide and 1.75 cm deep.[19] In general, each lobe is 'about the size and shape of half a plum cut vertically or about the size of the top segment of a person's thumb'.[4] Many women report that their thyroid enlarges slightly around each menstrual period and during pregnancy.[4]

A thin bridge called the isthmus (usually about 2 cm square and about 0.2–0.6 cm deep) connects the two lobes. However, up to

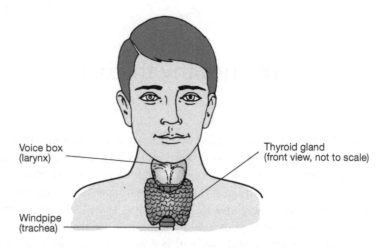

Voice box (larynx)

Thyroid gland (front view, not to scale)

Windpipe (trachea)

Figure 1.1 Position of the thyroid gland (not to scale)

1 in 25 people do not have an isthmus. A smooth 'coat', called the capsule, surrounds the gland. The thyroid receives a rich supply of blood and lymph. A 20 g thyroid receives about 5 litres of blood an hour – about half a bathtub's worth each day.[19]

Lymph

Lymph is a clear, yellowish fluid that bathes every part of your body and contains white blood cells, which help you fight infections. This is why your lymph nodes (such as the 'glands' under your chin and in your armpits) may swell when you have an infection. Lymph circulates through a network of vessels, called the lymphatic system, which collect fluid and proteins filtered from the blood. Lymph vessels return more than 4 litres of fluid back into the large veins in the neck every day. The liver and kidneys can then dispose of the waste fluids and proteins.

Retrosternal and substernal thyroids

Occasionally, part or all of the thyroid gland develops behind the breastbone (sternum):

- Retrosternal means that part of the gland is behind the breastbone (Figure 1.2).

- Substernal means that the entire thyroid is behind the breast-bone (Figure 1.3).

Provided the thyroid remains a healthy size, retrosternal and sub-sternal glands usually do not cause health problems. You may never know that the gland is misplaced. However, a growing misplaced

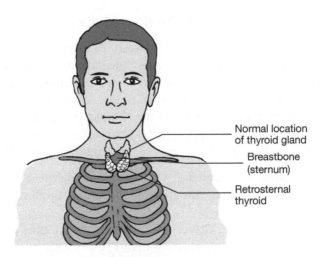

Normal location
of thyroid gland

Breastbone
(sternum)

Retrosternal
thyroid

Figure 1.2 Retrosternal thyroid gland

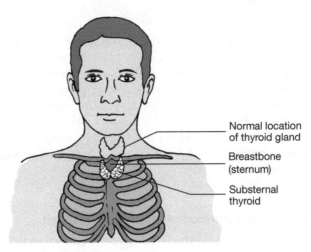

Normal location
of thyroid gland

Breastbone
(sternum)

Substernal
thyroid

Figure 1.3 Substernal thyroid gland

gland can squash the trachea, oesophagus (food pipe) and large veins in the neck. The limited space at the base of the neck around the top of the breastbone means that retrosternal glands are especially likely to cause problems. In rare cases, the thyroid develops in other parts of the throat – in about 9 of 10 cases, on or near the tongue. Doctors call these 'ectopic' thyroids.[20]

Inside the thyroid gland

Your thyroid gland contains between 20 million and 30 million microscopic spheres, called follicles,[6] surrounding a central core. This core is largely composed of a special protein called thyroglobulin. The gland can turn thyroglobulin into thyroid hormone. And thyroglobulin stores iodine, so the thyroid gland contains enough thyroid hormone to supply the body for up to 3 months.[18]

The follicle cells produce two types of thyroid hormone:[18]

- Thyroxine, also called T_4, contains four iodine atoms. About 80–90 per cent of the thyroid hormone produced by your thyroid is T_4.
- Triiodothyronine, also called T_3, carries three iodine atoms. T_3 is about four times more active than T_4.

What are hormones?

Hormones are a type of chemical messenger. (The term hormone comes from the Greek for 'I excite' or 'I arouse'.[21]) Your body produces 60 or so hormones, each of which has a specific action. Insulin, for instance, tells cells to take up more glucose (a type of sugar) from the blood as fuel. Oestrogen, progesterone and testosterone control reproduction. Adrenaline makes sure your body is ready to fight or run away from danger – biologists describe this as your level of arousal. As we will see, thyroid hormones also influence energy, reproduction and arousal. Thyroid diseases may be the most common hormone problem.[7]

Getting thyroid hormone to where it is needed

T_4 and T_3 move around the body transported by special proteins in the blood made by the liver, such as thyroxine-binding globulin (sometimes called thyroid-binding globulin), transthyretin and albumin. These proteins release thyroid hormone only where needed by your body. The hormone bound to the protein is inactive, which protects cells from overstimulation. In addition, transthyretin helps transport T_4 into the brain.[18]

The T_3 and T_4 that 'float' in the clear, watery, yellowish serum (essentially what remains when cells and several proteins in the blood form a clot) are responsible for the hormone's actions.[4] Almost every organ in your body – including muscle, the liver, kidney and brain – converts T_4 into T_3.[6] An enzyme (page x) removes one iodine atom to produce the T_3 that controls energy production by the cell. As mentioned earlier, T_3 is about four times more active than T_4.

A healthy person produces just enough thyroid hormone to meet their needs. Levels rise and fall according to the environment and the level of activity. The biological term is homeostasis: each cell, each tissue, each organism aims to compensate for internal and external changes and keep the body's critical functions within a narrow range. It's a bit like using a thermostat on a central heating system to keep the house at a comfortable temperature.

For example, when it's cold, thyroid hormone production rises. In response, cells convert more fuel to energy, which generates heat. Once you are warm, thyroid hormone production falls and cells convert less fuel to energy. Likewise, thyroid hormone levels rise during physical and mental stress to help you cope with the additional demands.[18]

Describing thyroid hormone and disease

Doctors use several terms to refer to thyroid hormone production and the associated changes in the body:

- Euthyroid describes normal thyroid hormone production.
- Hypothyroid refers to decreased production of thyroid hormone, which makes cells less active and, in some cases, too slow and sluggish to keep up with the demands on your body. Hypothyroidism can refer to thyroid underactivity even if the person does not develop symptoms or signs.
- Hyperthyroid refers to increased production of thyroid hormone, which makes the body's cells more active and, in some cases, go

into damaging overdrive. Hyperthyroidism can refer to over-activity of the thyroid even if the person does not develop symptoms or signs.

- Myxoedema refers to severe hypothyroidism, especially when the skin and underlying tissues swell, such as in thyroid eye disease (Chapter 6).
- Thyrotoxicosis describes the symptoms and signs caused by thyroid overactivity.
- Silent thyroiditis occurs when a virus or an autoimmune reaction produces symptoms, but does not cause any discomfort in the gland.[4]

The thyroid and your bones

In children, thyroid hormone stimulates the growth and development of several tissues, including the brain and skeleton.[18] Thyroid hormone also helps your skeleton repair wear and tear throughout your life.

Your skeleton might seem inert, but special cells constantly repair damaged or old areas. Your ankle, for instance, bears a force 1.5 times your body weight each time you take a step; running or jumping increases the force to some three or four times your body weight. In other words, damage is inevitable.

Specialized cells 'crawl' over your skeleton digging out old and damaged bone (resorption). Another group of cells lays down new bone. This process replaces all old or damaged bone in about 200 days, according to the National Osteoporosis Society.

Your thyroid gland helps balance bone breakdown and repair. Parafollicular cells (also called C cells) in the thyroid make a hormone called calcitonin. Bone breakdown releases calcium, and high levels of calcium in the blood trigger calcitonin release. In turn, calcitonin inhibits, for example, the cells that break down bone. Calcitonin also reduces the amount of calcium absorbed from food and drink as well as the amount of the mineral recycled by the kidneys. So blood levels of calcium return to normal. However, excessive calcitonin would inhibit the cells that break down damaged bone. High calcitonin levels hinder or prevent repair. So the body strikes another fine balance, in this case by releasing another hormone from another set of glands, called the parathyroids.

The parathyroid glands

The parathyroids are four small glands (3 × 6 mm) behind the thyroid gland, usually just inside the capsule (Figure 1.4). Occasionally, the parathyroids are embedded in the thyroid gland. When calcium levels are too low, the parathyroid glands release parathyroid hormone, which increases the production of new bone, the amount of calcium you absorb from food and the amount that the kidney recycles. This means that there is more calcium to use in making new bone.

An imbalance between calcitonin and parathyroid hormone may eventually weaken the skeleton and lead to osteoporosis (brittle bone disease). This means a minor bump or fall can break the bone – so-called fragility fractures – especially in the wrist and hip. The vertebrae in the spine may crumble or shrink, producing a rounded back, a hump and height loss.

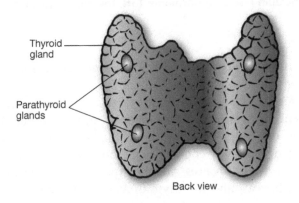

Back view

Figure 1.4 Position of the parathyroid glands

Controlling thyroid hormone levels

Your thyroid gland should tightly control hormone levels to meet, without exceeding, your body's energy demands. As a result, a network of signals controls the production and release of T_3 and T_4 using a mechanism known as a feedback loop (Figure 1.5 overleaf).

The signals begin in a part of the brain called the hypothalamus, which also helps control appetite. The hypothalamus produces, among other chemical messengers, thyrotropin-releasing hormone (TRH). When you feel cold or when levels of thyroid hormone fall,

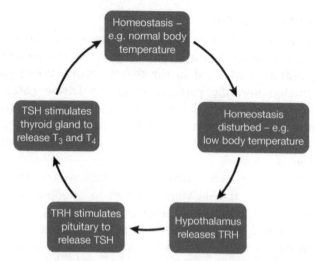

Figure 1.5 'Feedback loop' that controls thyroid hormone production (TRH, thyrotropin-releasing hormone; TSH, thyroid-stimulating hormone)

TRH levels rise.[18] As we will see later, appetite and body temperature often go awry in thyroid disease.

TRH travels to a gland behind the bridge of the nose – the pituitary. Depending on which doctor describes it, the pituitary is the size of a pea or a grape. The pituitary is the body's 'master' gland and directly or indirectly controls many other glands and organs, including the testes, ovaries, adrenals (page 141), milk production by the breasts, and the thyroid. As a result, some pituitary diseases cause thyroid problems, although these are relatively uncommon.

In response to TRH, the pituitary releases pulses of thyroid-stimulating hormone (TSH). Levels of TSH are higher by night than day, which helps ensure you have the thyroid hormone needed to meet the demands of the day. Levels can also change up to two- or threefold in healthy people over a year, partly to compensate for temperature variation and other seasonal changes.[4]

TSH stimulates the thyroid to release more T_3 and T_4. TSH also helps control the gland's growth and development, and stimulates the thyroid to increase iodine uptake. Indeed, levels of iodine in the thyroid gland are about 20–40 times higher than in the blood.[17]

When the hypothalamus detects high levels of thyroid hormone in the blood, or you feel warm, TRH production declines. In turn, the pituitary releases less TSH, and T_3 and T_4 levels therefore fall. This very sensitive feedback loop strictly controls the levels of T_3 and T_4 circulating around your body and, in turn, the speed of metabolism.[17] As we will see in Chapter 2, measuring TSH helps doctors assess how well your thyroid gland is working.

Receptors, drugs and the thyroid

Many of the body's chemical messengers, including TSH, work by binding to receptors. Graves' disease (see page 47), occurs when the immune system mistakenly stimulates TSH receptors. Some drugs

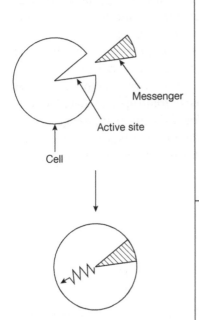

Messenger

Active site

Cell

The messenger binds to the active site, triggering the messages inside the cell that produce the biological effect

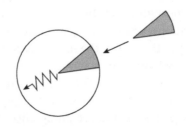

Agonists bind to the active site and trigger the messages, producing the same biological effect as the messenger

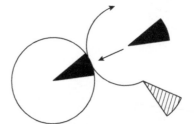

Antagonists bind to the active site and don't trigger the messages, but they prevent the messenger from binding, so blocking the biological effect

Figure 1.6 Drugs and receptors

used to treat thyroid disease also work by binding to receptors. So it's worth briefly introducing receptors (Figure 1.6 on the previous page).

Imagine a cell in the thyroid gland as a car. The receptor is the ignition. TSH (the messenger) is the key. When the key fits into the ignition lock, the engine starts. Likewise, when TSH binds to its receptor, part of the cell's internal machinery switches on. This effect is specific: just as your key only starts your car, the messenger only switches on those processes controlled by the receptor. TSH does not bind to and activate the receptor for insulin, for example.

Now imagine that you have a skeleton key. It also fits the ignition lock and switches on the engine. Some drugs act like a skeleton key. The receptor cannot distinguish the drug from the normal messenger (TSH). Both switch on the cell's machinery, acting as 'agonists'. For example, levothyroxine, used to treat hypothyroidism, binds to the same receptors and triggers the same responses as naturally produced thyroid hormone.

In other cases, the drug may fit the receptor, preventing the usual messenger from reaching the receptor, but does not switch on the cell's machinery. These drugs are 'antagonists'. Doctors may treat certain symptoms caused by hyperthyroidism with beta-blockers (page 58). These are antagonists for a chemical messenger called noradrenaline. Normally, noradrenaline increases your heart rate and blood pressure. So beta-blockers reduce heart rate and blood pressure.

2

Testing your thyroid

The signs and symptoms produced by the various thyroid diseases are often vague, usually subjective and, in many cases, ambiguous. For example, people with hypothyroidism may report fatigue, aching muscles and constipation.[22] However, you may be tired because your blood sugar levels are too low, you have an infection or had a bad night's sleep. Your muscles may ache because you are worn out, worked too hard at the gym or took certain drugs, such as some of those that lower cholesterol (page 102). Constipation is often a sign you are not eating enough fibre (page 103), not drinking enough fluids, have irritable bowel syndrome (page 35) or another disease. And constipation is common: a Danish study found that 39 per cent of 373 patients had constipation when admitted to hospital.[23]

Likewise, anxiety, irritability, nervousness, difficulty sleeping and changes in libido do not necessarily indicate an overactive thyroid gland. They can be signs of stress – either in general or because you carry the burden of living with a serious disease. Some people with hyperthyroidism experience constant thirst and urinate a lot – similar symptoms to diabetes.[7]

As a result, doctors use a variety of tests to assess how well your thyroid is working. Indeed, thyroid testing is routine. In any year, between 18 and 25 per cent of people visiting their GP have their thyroid function tested for several reasons, including weight gain, depression, tiredness, menstrual irregularities or during a health screen.[5] In part, widespread testing and increasingly sensitive tests explain the rise in the number of people diagnosed with thyroid disease. Yet subtle and ambiguous signs and symptoms mean that many people probably never see their GP. Their thyroid problems go undiagnosed and they suffer unnecessarily.

Signs and symptoms

In addition to asking about your symptoms, doctors will look for signs of thyroid disease:

- Symptoms are changes that you experience. These can be obvious, such as hair loss, goitre (Chapter 3) or changes to your eyes (Chapter 6). Other symptoms, such as anxiety, depression and pain, are not directly on show but may change your behaviour.
- Signs are changes that doctors can measure, such as blood pressure, heart rate or levels of TSH (page 13) in your blood. You can have an abnormal sign without feeling ill; for example, dangerously raised blood pressure (hypertension), high concentrations of cholesterol or low TSH levels. That is why it is so important to take your medicines whether or not you feel unwell.

Doctors base about 80 per cent of diagnoses on what patients reveal. However, Andrew Russell comments (see 'Further reading') that when questioned after seeing their GP, about 60 per cent of patients had not disclosed some symptoms during the consultation because, for example, they felt asking was inappropriate, feared a bad reaction or felt hurried. Your doctor cannot diagnose and treat you appropriately without the full picture.

However, recalling all the symptoms can be hard, and you may not accurately remember how they waxed and waned. So some people with thyroid disease keep a diary recording their weight, pulse and physical changes. They note whether they feel hot or cold, tired or full of beans, happy and relaxed or anxious and depressed, and so on. A long-term record helps you measure changes produced by conventional or complementary therapy, makes it easier for the doctor to assess your condition and helps you exert a sense of control over your thyroid disease. Nevertheless, try not to become obsessed with recording how you feel: you are more than a collection of comments or columns of figures.

Try to be specific when describing your symptoms. Rather than telling the doctor 'my eyes are sore', describe whether it feels like grittiness, pain or double vision when you look in a particular direction.[7] Likewise, if you complain vaguely of a sore throat and your tonsils or the back of your throat are pinker than the doctor would expect, your GP may miss subacute viral thyroiditis (page 93). You need to make clear exactly where your neck is sore. Discomfort in the front of the neck helps guide the doctor towards the thyroid.[4]

Thyroid function tests

Over the past few years, technological advances have allowed doctors to measure smaller and smaller amounts of T_3, T_4 and TSH (page 8). Modern thyroid function tests are exquisitely sensitive and invaluable aids to diagnosis, and help track how well you respond to treatment. However, thyroid function tests do not identify the specific underlying problem.[24]

For example, many people who complain of symptoms that could indicate thyroid disease have normal levels of 'free' T_4 and TSH. Normal blood levels of TSH essentially rule out thyroid disease in otherwise healthy people.[25] However, diseases affecting the pituitary gland or hypothalamus occasionally produce 'secondary' hypothyroidism. In these cases, people develop symptoms of hypothyroidism despite normal levels of TSH.

'Free' T_4 refers to the levels 'floating' in the serum and available to cells, rather than the proportion bound to transport proteins (page 4). A normal free T_4 level excludes secondary hypothyroidism. So if your TSH and free T_4 levels are normal, and you do not have another illness and are not taking drugs that can influence thyroid function, another disease is probably responsible for your symptoms.[24,25]

TSH: A window onto the thyroid

Modern highly sensitive TSH tests allow doctors to diagnose almost every case of thyroid disease. As we saw in Chapter 1, T_4 levels in the blood control the release of TSH from the pituitary. So:

- In hyperthyroidism, high T_4 levels reduce TSH production.
- In hypothyroidism, low levels of T_4 trigger a marked rise in TSH levels.[6]

These changes in TSH levels compensate for altered thyroid hormone production.[4]

Ever more sensitive tests introduced in recent years allow doctors to detect very subtle changes in TSH and T_4 levels. So they increasingly diagnose mild ('subclinical') thyroid disease. In subclinical hyper- or hypothyroidism, TSH levels fall and rise, respectively, while T_4 levels remain normal.

Subclinical hypo- or hyperthyroidism may never develop into full-blown (overt) thyroid disease. For example, between a quarter and three-quarters of people with subclinical hyperthyroidism no longer show abnormal readings when retested weeks or months later. In some people, the body repairs the damage. In others, non-thyroid diseases, drugs and diet triggered the subclinical hyperthyroidism.[26] Likewise, TSH levels returned to normal in more than a third (37 per cent) of people with subclinical hypothyroidism after an average of 32 months.[8] As a result, doctors often diagnose hyper- or hypothyroidism only if TSH levels do not return to normal after several weeks or months.

Measuring T_4 and T_3 levels

As mentioned in Chapter 1, most thyroid hormone circulates in the blood attached to proteins. The body cannot use this 'bound' thyroid hormone. Cells convert free T_4 into T_3. In other words, free T_4 indirectly indicates levels of thyroid hormone that the body can use.

However, numerous factors can change levels of total T_3, T_4 or both (see Table 2.1). For example, women taking contraceptives or hormone replacement therapy containing oestrogen, as well as those who are pregnant, produce more of the proteins that carry thyroid hormone (page 4). In response, total T_4 levels rise. However, the woman does not develop overt hyperthyroidism because the amount of free T_4 remains normal. Aspirin and many other drugs also bind to the carrier proteins. As a result, total T_4 levels fall. Again, free levels remain normal.[4] In other words, free T_4 seems to offer the best indication of your thyroid's health.

Measuring T_3 levels can offer additional insights. Levels of T_3 and T_4 usually move in parallel. However, in some people with hyperthyroidism, T_3 levels increase several weeks or months before T_4 changes. Occasionally, only T_3 levels increase in people with thyrotoxicosis. Conversely, several physical and mental illnesses unrelated to the thyroid gland can reduce T_3 levels. In these cases, T_3 levels return to normal after the underlying illness has passed.[4]

Once the doctor confirms that you have thyroid disease and starts treatment, you will need regular blood tests to see how well the management is working and to adjust the dose and drugs

Table 2.1 Factors that alter total T_4 or T_3 or both

Factors that increase total T_4 or T_3 or both include:

Pregnancy

Contraceptive pill, hormone replacement therapy (HRT) and other medicines containing oestrogen

Amiodarone – used to treat heart arrhythmias

Clofibrate – used to reduce high levels of cholesterol and other fats in the blood

Phenothiazines (e.g. chlorpromazine) – used to treat schizophrenia and some other serious mental illnesses

Carrying genes that increase levels of thyroxine-binding globulin

Factors that reduce total T_4 or T_3 or both include:

Kidney disease and other conditions that reduce levels of protein in the blood

Acromegaly – caused by excessive production of growth hormone by the pituitary gland

Cushing's syndrome – caused by high levels of steroids in the body, either as treatment for inflammatory disease or because of very high levels of a hormone called cortisol

Carrying genes that reduce levels of thyroxine-binding globulin (or the protein is absent)

Phenylbutazone – very occasionally used for ankylosing spondylitis, a type of arthritis in the spine

Phenytoin – used to treat epilepsy

Aspirin

Some antidepressants

Source: Adapted from Vanderpump and Tunbridge[4]

accordingly. Once you are on a stable treatment, you may need blood tests less often: the frequency depends on your particular circumstances. Nevertheless, it is important that you do not miss an appointment. Your doctor needs to assess your thyroid function to ensure that you are receiving the appropriate dose and type of treatment. And always let your doctor know if you develop symptoms between scheduled blood tests.

Are you normal?

Doctors define whether your thyroid is under- or overactive by comparing your results to a 'reference' or 'normal' range, produced by testing a large number of people. However, some people argue that a healthy level of thyroid hormones depends on the person, and that the ranges used by doctors may not apply to everyone. Therefore, unless you underwent a thyroid function test when you were healthy, it is difficult to know whether the reading is abnormal for you.[7] Indeed, the signs and symptoms that can arise from sub-clinical thyroid disease raise the question of whether these ranges really are 'normal'.[7] But doctors have little else to base treatment on other than the reference range. However, if you still experience symptoms of thyroid disease despite the blood tests giving your gland a clean bill of health, it is worth persisting. A trial of medicine may settle the case.

Body temperature and self-diagnosis

Heat is a by-product of metabolism. If your metabolism is sluggish, your body temperature may fall. If it is overactive, your temperature may rise. In healthy people, body temperature is highest while you are awake and lowest while you are asleep. Some self-help books for thyroid disease suggest measuring your body temperature every morning. Normal body temperature varies from 36.6°C (97.8°F) to 36.8°C (98.2°F). A temperature over 38°C (100.4°F) usually means you have a fever. If your body temperature is persistently low, you might have an underactive thyroid. However, body temperature varies for numerous reasons. In other words, while measuring your body temperature may help diagnosis, it is not definitive.[27]

Antibody tests

As mentioned earlier in this chapter, measuring levels of TSH and free T_4 does not identify the cause of the problem.[24] Therefore, doctors will look at the pattern of signs and symptoms, and perform other tests to see what's wrong.

For example, some thyroid diseases arise when the body's immune system mistakenly attacks the gland (see page 48). A group of pro-teins called autoantibodies allows the immune system to 'home in' on the thyroid. So doctors may test for autoantibodies against thyroid peroxidase – an enzyme critical for the normal production of thyroid hormone. Autoantibodies targeting thyroid peroxidase destroy the gland over several years. Testing for this antibody aids diagnosis of Hashimoto's thyroiditis (page 40).

Autoantibodies against the TSH receptor can cause Graves' disease (page 47). Some people with Graves' disease also develop antibodies against thyroid peroxidase or thyroglobulin. In these cases, the antibodies are part of a general autoimmune attack on the gland.[4]

Currently, we do not have any treatments that halt the auto-immune destruction of the thyroid. However, tracking the disease allows doctors to optimize therapy to slow its progression and alle-viate the symptoms. Antibody tests can also differentiate some of the main causes of thyroiditis:

- Infection (page 92)
- After giving birth (postpartum – page 86)
- Autoimmune damage.

Viral and postpartum thyroiditis usually resolve once the inflamma-tion subsides. However, autoimmune thyroiditis can permanently damage the gland. Nevertheless, autoantibodies alone do not clinch the diagnosis. For example, you may develop antibodies, but the damage may not be widespread enough to cause symptoms. At least 20 per cent of women aged over 50 years show antibodies against thyroid peroxidase. However, their thyroid function tests are normal.[22]

Spotting thyroid disease

Thyroid autoimmunity seems to be linked to acne in women, Greek researchers reported during the 2013 European Association of Dermatology and Venereology Congress in Istanbul. The 107 women with acne in the study were more likely to express high levels of antibodies against thyroglobulin (page 4) than 60 healthy women. This 'predilection for thyroid autoimmunity' may suggest that it's worth evaluating the thyroid function of adult women with acne.

Ultrasound scanning

Ultrasound scanners bounce sound waves off tissue. Differences in the strength of the signal as it returns to the machine construct a picture of the tissue – it's the same process used to look at a devel-oping baby during pregnancy. Ultrasonography can painlessly image the thyroid gland and the surrounding structures in the neck and chest. Doctors may, for example, suggest an ultrasound scan to see whether you have one or several thyroid nodules (lumps of tissue; Chapter 3).[8] Modern ultrasound systems can detect nodules just 2–3 mm across.[28] Ultrasonography may also detect whether the nodule is solid or a fluid-filled cyst. However, it cannot distinguish benign (non-malignant) from cancerous nodules.

Futhermore, as more people have ultrasound scans for a variety of ailments, doctors are discovering that between a quarter and a half of adults develop thyroid nodules.[29] About 90 per cent of thyroid nodules do not need treatment. Nevertheless, your doctor may suggest monitoring the nodule to watch for changes in size or other characteristics that could suggest it is becoming malignant.[29]

Your doctor might also suggest a CT or MRI scan. For example, a scan may help to confirm that you have thyroid eye disease (Chapter 6) if, for example, only one eye changes. A scan can also ascertain whether the swollen tissue around the eye is pressing on the optic nerve, which carries messages to the brain from the light-sensitive retina covering the back of the eye, before it begins to affect your vision.[4]

Thyroid biopsy

Sometimes, the only way to diagnose which thyroid disease you have is to take a small sample using a very thin needle, a procedure called fine-needle aspiration biopsy (FNAB) or fine-needle aspiration cytology (cytology means the study of cells).

The British Thyroid Foundation says that most people describe FNAB as about as uncomfortable as having a blood sample taken. But if you find FNAB very unpleasant or are very anxious, your doctor might offer a local anaesthetic (for example as a cream) to numb the area. Taking paracetamol an hour before FNAB might also help, especially if the doctor needs to sample more than one nodule.[30]

Doctors examine the biopsy under a microscope and use a variety of other tests, such as looking for hallmark changes in certain proteins, to determine whether a nodule is cancerous. Chapter 7 looks at the various types of thyroid cancer and their treatment. Unfortunately, the results of FNAB are not definitive in up to 30 per cent of samples, and up to 1 in 5 aspirations yield an inadequate sample. In such cases, you will probably need a second FNAB.[4]

Researchers are also beginning to characterize the hallmark changes in genes (page 25) and other proteins that drive the growth and development of thyroid cancer. In the near future, doctors will probably look for these alterations ('biomarkers') to distinguish thyroid cancer from benign nodules.[29] Another new test – called elastography – measures a nodule's hardness, which depends on whether it is malignant or benign.[28] However, at the time of writing, further studies are needed before these tests are used routinely.

Radioactive iodine scan

If blood tests suggest that your thyroid is overactive, your doctor may suggest a radioactive iodine (radioiodine) scan. You swallow a small amount of radioiodine and then return a few hours later or the next day. The dose of radiation is much less than that used to treat hyperthyroidism or thyroid cancer (Chapter 7).

A camera that is sensitive to radiation scans the thyroid from different angles. An overactive area takes up more radioiodine than a healthy region. Doctors call this a 'hot' area. As the hot nodule pumps out massive amounts of thyroid hormone, the feedback loop (page 8) suppresses production elsewhere in the gland. As a result, underactive, 'cold', areas take up less iodine than healthy tissue.

This pattern of 'hot' and 'cold' areas offers other clues to the cause of the thyroid disease:

- In Graves' disease, the entire thyroid appears overactive. Scans show high, but evenly spread, activity across both lobes, which are usually enlarged.
- In multinodular toxic goitre, the scan shows several 'islands of activity' that differ in size and the intensity of the 'heat', separated by cold areas.[4]
- An overactive thyroid triggered by a viral infection or a 'silent' autoimmune attack (in other words, one that does not cause signs or symptoms) can temporarily stop working. As a result, the entire gland appears 'cold'.[4]

Using a variety of tests, taking a medical history and looking at your pattern of signs and symptoms, doctors can diagnose most causes of thyroid disease. However, you must be honest with your doctors to allow them to gain a full picture of your physical and mental symptoms, as well as the impact that the thyroid disease is having on your quality of life and ability to take part in normal day-to-day activities.

3

Goitres and nodules

Goitres are probably the best-known and most characteristic of the changes caused by thyroid disease. A goitre can range from only slightly larger than usual (about 20 g in an adult)[19] to 'the size of an orange or even larger' (Figure 3.1).[4] One goitre left a man with a neck size of 60 cm. (Some people first notice a goitre when they cannot do up the top button of a blouse or shirt.) When surgeons removed the goitre, it weighed 700 g.[1] Try searching for 'massive goitre' on the internet – but it's not for the overly squeamish.

As we saw in the Introduction, up to 80 per cent of people in areas with severely low levels of iodine developed goitres before the mineral was widely added to food.[8] Low iodine levels meant that the thyroid needed to work harder. In response, the gland expanded to capture sufficient iodine from the blood. Goitres can also arise from excessive iodine intake or hyperthyroidism. The excessive hormone production overstimulates and enlarges the gland.

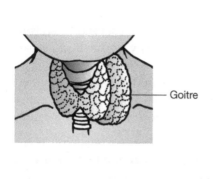
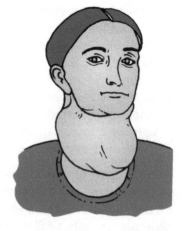

Goitre

Figure 3.1 Goitres

A common problem

Goitres remain common, even in countries where public health officials believe that most people get the iodine they need from their diets. A UK study, for example, found that 15.5 per cent of adults had goitres that doctors could detect by touching their throat.[2] A goitre needs to be at least 10 mm across before a doctor can feel the enlargement.[19]

Sometimes (especially in premenopausal women[8]), the whole gland increases in size, called a 'simple diffuse' goitre. The doctor will test for cancer and autoimmune diseases that can also cause diffuse goitre, such as Hashimoto's thyroiditis (page 40) and Graves' disease (page 47).

Sometimes only one area gets bigger – a solitary nodule. Sometimes several discrete areas enlarge – 'multinodular' goitres. However, most nodules are so tiny that they are seen only on an ultrasound scan, which can detect nodules between 1 and 2 mm across. Ultrasonography reveals at least one additional nodule in up to half of people with a single nodule that the doctor can feel.[31] In one study, 56 per cent of 369 people without thyroid cancer had nodules greater than 5 mm on ultrasound. About a third had more than one nodule, while 8 and 9 per cent had three and four nodules, respectively.[32] In other words, multinodular goitres may be more common than doctors have traditionally believed.

Types of multinodular goitre

Multinodular goitres tend to arise from low-level and, probably, intermittent stimulus to the thyroid gland from, for example, low levels of iodine, goitrogens in the diet (page 105), or an auto-immune disease that promotes clusters of cells to multiply. Some nodules arise from a simple non-toxic goitre.[4]

Multinodular goitres may contain colloid nodules – excessive growth of normal tissue – which doctors can usually identify using ultrasound scanning and FNAB (page 18). According to the British Thyroid Foundation, colloid nodules may not need treatment if they do not cause symptoms or are not unsightly. FNAB can rule out thyroid cancer. Often doctors will sample the largest ('dominant') nodule. However, this assumes that the other nodules are benign. Therefore, if you decide against treatment it is still worth keeping an eye on your thyroid.

Other nodules ('hyperplastic' nodules) look like a cancer on an ultrasound scan and FNAB, but are often benign. Doctors may suggest removing hyperplastic nodules, which can be solitary or multinodular, to be on the safe side. Experts at the hospital will then examine the nodule to see if it was malignant. Whether the nodule was benign or malignant influences your future management.

Toxic and non-toxic goitres

A large goitre does not necessarily produce excessive amounts of thyroid hormone. A large, poorly functioning goitre may still cause hypothyroidism. Conversely, a small goitre may produce excessive amounts of thyroid hormone.[4] As a result, doctors describe goitres as either 'toxic' or 'non-toxic'.

Toxic goitres make too much thyroid hormone.[2] Toxic multi-nodular goitres usually arise in people aged between 50 and 70. These people typically report that their goitre gradually enlarged and became lumpy over several years. The signs and symptoms of hyperthyroidism develop slowly. In some people, the signs and symptoms resemble Graves' disease. In some, heart failure is the first indication that the goitre has produced hypothyroidism (page 31).[4] Overall, up to a quarter of people with multinodular goitre develop overt or subclinical hyperthyroidism.[31]

Benign tumours can form solitary toxic nodules, which can take over hormone production for the entire gland. As a result, the rest of the cells that produce thyroid hormone become inactive and appear cold on a radioiodine scan.[4]

Nodules and thyroid cancer

Although nodules are not usually malignant, you should get any nodules or goitres checked as soon as possible:

- Thyroid adenoma is a non-cancerous growth. Many continue to expand and so surgeons often suggest removal. The hospital will check the adenoma to make sure that it is not cancerous.
- A thyroid cyst is a fluid-filled swelling. An ultrasound scan (page 17) usually distinguishes a cyst from other types of nodule.

Surgeons can usually drain the fluid using a fine needle. However, if this does not work you may need more invasive surgery.

The British Thyroid Foundation notes that unless they grow rapidly, multinodular goitres are rarely cancerous, although it is always worth checking. In particular, make sure that your doctor checks any nodule that grows over a few weeks or if you develop high-pitched wheezing (stridor), hoarseness or swelling of the lymph glands around the neck.[16]

Large nodules are not necessarily more likely to be cancerous than smaller lumps.[28] The increasing sensitivity of imaging allows doctors to detect tiny malignancies. For example, up to a third of adults show small (less than 1 cm) 'microcarcinomas'.[8] Many of these microcarcinomas are too small and grow too slowly to cause symptoms. If a scan for thyroid disease or another illness reveals microcarcinomas, you will need to discuss the risks and benefits of treatment with your doctor, especially if you are older. Put rather bluntly: you may be more likely to die before the cancer causes any problem. However, you will live knowing you have cancer, which some people find stressful. Chapter 7 looks at thyroid cancer.

Causes of goitres and nodules

Goitres and thyroid nodules arise from the interaction between genetic (page 25) and environmental factors. For example, on average, about 1 in 1,000 people develop thyroid nodules each year.[28] The rate increases to about 1 in 50 among people exposed to radiation during childhood (such as following a nuclear accident) or at work.[28] Radiotherapy (X-ray treatment) to the head and neck, for example for cancer, can also trigger nodules.

However, even a healthy diet and normal life events may be risk factors for goitres. For example, pearl millet and soy can inhibit thyroid peroxidase (page 16). Cassava, sweet potato, sorghum and cruciferous vegetables (such as cabbage, cauliflower, broccoli and turnips) contain chemicals that can reduce the amount of iodine that the thyroid takes up from blood.[2] Doctors describe these goitre-promoting foods as goitrogens. Patsy Westcott advises limiting your intake of foods that can reduce iodine uptake (page 105) if you have hypothyroidism.[7]

Goitres are also especially common during pregnancy and around the menopause. So hormones probably contribute to some goitres and nodules. A UK study found that women were about 4.5 times more likely to develop goitre than men.[2] We will see this pattern time and again: women are much more likely to develop thyroid diseases than men. Nevertheless, in many cases doctors may not be able to pinpoint a cause.

What is a risk factor?

A risk factor increases your chance of developing a particular disease. For example, smoking is a risk factor for many cancers; dangerously high blood pressure (hypertension) is a risk factor for stroke; and excessive alcohol consumption is a risk factor for liver disease. However, having one or more risk factors does not mean that the disease is inevitable – everyone seems to have a relative who smoked, ate an unhealthy diet and drank heavily and yet died at a ripe old age. You may also develop the disease without having a common risk factor: according to Cancer Research UK, 14 per cent of lung cancers were not caused by active or passive smoking.

But not everyone exposed to radiation, not every mum-to-be, not everyone in parts of the world where millet or seaweed is a staple food develops goitre. Even in parts of the world where it is endemic, at least a fifth of people do not have goitres. So it factors contribute – and many of these are in your genes.

For example, children of people with goitres are more likely to develop the swelling themselves, irrespective of the amount of iodine in their diet. Several other thyroid diseases seem to run in families, although the signs and symptoms can change through the generations: one family member may have hypothyroidism, another hyperthyroidism. In some cases, the thyroid disease seems to skip a generation.[4] However, in the past, doctors may have missed subclinical disease, giving the impression that some generations had avoided thyroid disease.

Today, researchers recognize that several genes interact to determine the risk of goitres and other thyroid diseases. Some genes predispose to thyroid disease. Others protect. The balance of genes children inherit from their biological parents interacts with the environment. And it's this interaction that determines the likelihood they will develop thyroid disease.

Genes and thyroid disease

Almost every one of your 10 trillion cells contains an 'instruction manual' to make your entire body, encoded in DNA's famous double helix.

The amount of DNA in your body almost defies belief. According to the leading science journal *Nature*, your DNA – pulled into a single, microscopically thin strand – would go from Earth to the Sun and back more than 300 times, or encircle the Earth's equator 2.5 million times.[33]

In humans, DNA is tightly wrapped into 23 chromosomes that contain the 25,000 or so genes that make you 'you'. You get almost half your genes from your father and the rest from your mother. (If you are wondering why it is not quite half, the genes for mitochondria – the cell's powerhouses – always come from the mother.) These genes determine the colour of your eyes and hair, your features and your chances of developing certain diseases.

Each gene tells the cell to make one or more proteins. Cells can modify the proteins produced by the gene: for example, chopping some into smaller versions or joining others together. This means we can make more proteins than we have genes.

Typically, several proteins participate in every biological process that keeps us alive. So we need a staggering number. Bill Bryson notes that humans may produce between 200,000 and a million different proteins. Indeed, each cell may produce more than 10,000 different proteins.[34]

The genes that make these proteins switch on (beginning a process called transcription, which produces the protein) and off depending on the body's needs and the cell's role. In a healthy thyroid gland, a gene in the follicle makes a protein needed by the follicle, rather than one for the tongue, eye or even a C cell.

Faults in genes or the processes controlling transcription can also tell the body to make too much or too little of a critical protein. You might produce high or low levels of the proteins that carry thyroid hormone around the body, which influences your blood tests. Faulty genes may also cause thyroid hormone resistance, where the receptors on cells in organs around the body do not respond properly to thyroid hormone. Furthermore, several genes control the pathways that make T_3 and T_4. If one of these genes is faulty, people do not produce enough thyroid hormone. Goitres arise as the gland tries to compensate.[4] However, these are very rare and we will not consider these diseases further.

Treating goitres

Patients with goitres may see their doctor because the swelling is unsightly or causes unpleasant symptoms.[2] For example:

- A large goitre can press on the oesophagus. This can make swallowing uncomfortable and even cause choking.
- A goitre may create a sensation of pressure or pain in your neck, especially when you lie down.
- A very large goitre can press on the trachea, possibly causing breathing difficulties (including stridor, shortness of breath, or pain), particularly when exercising.
- The goitre can compress the nerves supplying the larynx (voice box). This may result in a hoarse, weak voice.
- A large goitre may press on the veins carrying blood from the face and brain back to the heart. This increases the amount of blood in your head, leaving you with a feeling of fullness in your head.[4]

Retrosternal or substernal goitres (page 3), in particular, may squeeze the trachea or oesophagus, blood vessels or other surrounding tissue.[28] Your doctor may suggest a scan to confirm this. Goitres and nodules that cause symptoms usually need treatment and you will need to balance the risks and benefits of each approach.

Surgery

Surgeons can cut away part or all of the thyroid gland to remove the goitre or nodule – an operation called thyroidectomy. In general, surgeons make the incision in one of the natural creases in the skin of the neck. Once the initial redness fades, most scars are fine lines that are indistinguishable from a natural crease. I worked with someone regularly for 2 years, sitting directly opposite or next to her at meetings, before I realized that she had undergone an operation on her thyroid. Even then, she had to tell me. The scar was almost invisible, even when she pointed it out and I peered closely. Nevertheless, while the cosmetic appearance is generally very good, doctors may not be able to guarantee that it will be.[4]

Between 2 and 5 per cent of people develop complications after thyroid surgery, including hypothyroidism. For example, a study of 3,574 thyroid operations reported damage to the nerve controlling the larynx in about 2 per cent of cases, and underactivity of the parathyroid glands (page 7) in around 3 per cent.[35] Furthermore, if the surgeon does not remove the entire gland – an operation called subtotal thyroidectomy – about 60 per cent of multinodular goitres eventually recur.[2] Therefore, it is a good idea to ask what the complication and success rates are for any hospital and surgeon. However, bear in mind that the best surgeons tend to get the most difficult cases. Furthermore, people with difficult cases are inherently more likely to develop complications and the success rates are usually lower.

Levothyroxine

Levothyroxine (see page 42) offers an alternative to surgery for some non-toxic multinodular goitres that arise to compensate for reduced production of thyroid hormone. Levothyroxine 'tops up' the missing thyroid hormone. In some cases, your doctor may suggest combining levothyroxine and iodine supplements. As the gland does not need to work as hard, the goitre shrinks.

Taking levothyroxine for between 6 and 12 months typically reduces goitre size by 20–40 per cent. However, the goitre usually returns to its pretreatment size if you stop taking levothyroxine. So you may need to take levothyroxine for the rest of your life.[2] You will also need to take levothyroxine if a surgeon removes most or all of your thyroid gland.

Radioiodine

Radioiodine offers another treatment for toxic multinodular goitres. As mentioned in Chapter 2, a hot nodule suppresses the activity of other cells in the gland. As a result, hot nodules take up more radioiodine than the rest of the gland. In turn, radioiodine specifically destroys the hot nodules. The healthy thyroid tissue gradually returns to normal.[4]

Indeed, some doctors regard radioiodine as the treatment of choice for most toxic adenomas and multinodular goitres.[24] Other doctors prefer to reserve radioiodine for special cases, such as when surgery is especially risky.

The thyroid concentrates the radioactive mineral, which limits the collateral damage to healthy tissue in the rest of your body. However, about 30 per cent of people develop hypothyroidism after receiving radioiodine.[2]

Radioiodine's full effects take about 2–3 months to emerge,[4] but may halve the size of non-toxic multinodular goitres after a year.[2] By contrast, levothyroxine begins reducing the goitre's size within a week or two.[4]

The radioactivity decays over a few weeks. In the meantime, your doctor will suggest avoiding close (for example, less than a metre) and prolonged (usually more than an hour) contact with other people – especially children and pregnant women – for up to 4 weeks after receiving radioiodine.[4] Avoiding contact may be difficult if, for example, you have young children. The exact time depends on your individual circumstances, so make sure you fully understand any restrictions.

Clearly, you need to discuss the advantages and disadvantages of each approach with your doctor and, perhaps, speak to a patient support group. However, modern treatments allow doctors to treat most goitres safely and effectively.

4

Hypothyroidism

Hypothyroidism occurs when an underactive thyroid gland does not produce enough hormone to meet your body's needs. Some people don't develop signs and symptoms. But many people find that their metabolism becomes sluggish and they develop unpleasant and sometimes debilitating symptoms. Indeed, according to Stephen Langer and James Scheer in *Solved: The Riddle of Illness*, hypothyroidism causes 'more than 64 symptoms'. In *Why am I so Tired?*, Martin Budd puts the figure even higher: more than '100 symptoms [are] caused by thyroid deficiency'.

Whatever the exact figure, the symptoms of hypothyroidism are a very mixed bag, ranging from mild fatigue or modest anxiety to a profoundly disturbed mental state and the thankfully very rare, but potentially fatal myxoedema coma. This symptomatic diversity can make hypothyroidism difficult to diagnose, especially as the severity might not directly reflect the biochemical findings – a paradox illustrated by subclinical hypothyroidism.

Subclinical hypothyroidism

As mentioned in Chapter 2, doctors diagnose hypothyroidism biochemically when TSH levels are high and T_4 levels are low, after ruling out other possible causes. At first, however, TSH levels usually rise, while concentrations of free T_4 and free T_3 remain normal. The increase in TSH compensates for the gland's underactivity. Doctors call this 'subclinical' hypothyroidism.

Subclinical hypothyroidism is relatively common. A study from north-east England found that 8 per cent of women and 10 per cent of those over 55 years of age had subclinical hypothyroidism. As is usually the case with thyroid disease, women are much more likely to develop this ailment: 3 per cent of men had subclinical hypothyroidism.[8]

Subclinical hypothyroidism is something of a misnomer. Usually, subclinical implies that the person does not exhibit symptoms or signs. However, up to a quarter of people with subclinical hypothyroidism detected by biochemical testing develop symptoms caused by an underactive thyroid gland,[24] including dry skin, cold intolerance and fatigue.[4]

Subclinical hypothyroidism and the heart

In addition, some, but not all, studies link subclinical hypothyroidism to an increased risk of developing cardiovascular (heart and blood vessels) disease:

- People with subclinical hypothyroidism tend to show higher blood pressure than those without thyroid disease.[25] Hypertension increases the risk of strokes, heart attacks and other serious diseases.
- Some people with subclinical hypothyroidism show increased levels of cholesterol in their blood (page 36), especially if, for example, they smoke or show early signs of diabetes (insulin resistance).[25] Again, raised levels of cholesterol increase the risk of stroke, heart attacks and so on.
- Subclinical hypothyroidism may increase the risk of heart failure, especially in elderly people. However, some studies failed to find a link between subclinical hypothyroidism and heart failure.[25] Nevertheless, heart failure is common even in people without thyroid disease. So it is a good idea to know the signs and symptoms.

Further studies are needed to clarify the relationship between subclinical hypothyroidism and both heart disease and deaths from cardiovascular causes. However, based on the evidence at the time of writing, subclinical hypothyroidism *might* increase the risk of cardiovascular problems by up to 50 per cent in people over 65 years of age.[25] Subclinical hypothyroidism *might* also increase the risk of heart attacks and death from cardiovascular disease.[6] Clearly, reducing your risk of heart disease by, for example, quitting smoking, exercising and eating healthily is still sensible.

What is heart failure?

Each year, around 27,000 people in the UK learn that they have developed heart failure, caused by the heart failing to pump enough blood to meet the body's demands. Doctors divide heart failure into left and right forms. Eventually, most people with heart failure develop both to a greater or lesser extent. In left heart failure, the left ventricle (page 53) cannot pump enough of the blood that it receives from the lungs. So blood backs up in the lungs, causing breathlessness. This is potentially fatal. In right heart failure, the right ventricle cannot pump enough of the blood received from the body. As a result, blood backs up in the legs, ankles, torso and so on, causing peripheral oedema (congestion – which is why doctors refer to this problem as congestive heart failure). This oedema is usually uncomfortable and may produce skin ulcers.

Subclinical hypothyroidism and the brain

Your brain accounts for about 2 per cent of your body weight – it weighs about 1.3–1.4 kg (3 lb) – but uses around 20 per cent of the glucose in your blood. The blood flow to the brain seems to decline in people with hypothyroidism. Meanwhile, the fall in thyroid hormone means that the brain converts less glucose to energy. These changes might help explain why people with overt and subclinical hypothyroidism are especially likely to develop psychological problems, especially depression and anxiety (see Chapter 11).[22,24,35]

Some people with subclinical hypothyroidism exhibit mental changes, including cognitive impairment – a reduction in, for example, the ability to think clearly, remember things and solve problems. You may lose keys and shopping lists, miss appointments or forget where you parked your car. In some cases, these mental changes may mimic age-related memory loss or even be so profound that they are mistaken for dementia.

We all have memory lapses from time to time. However, it is worth seeing your doctor if you feel your memory is worse than it used to be, you feel mentally 'cloudy' or depression or anxiety is making your life miserable. Do not be tempted to write the symptoms off as a sign of ageing or stress.

Treating and monitoring subclinical hypothyroidism

Many doctors believe that subclinical hypothyroidism does not need treatment unless you have symptoms, are pregnant, are trying to have a baby or have heart failure.[25] So if the only sign is a rise in TSH levels, your doctor may suggest monitoring your thyroid function to detect whether the disease advances to overt hypothyroidism.

Subclinical hypothyroidism does not inevitably lead to the full-blown disease. In one study, 37 per cent of cases of subclinical hypothyroidism had resolved after an average of 32 months.[25] However, each year, 5 per cent of people with high levels of TSH *and* autoantibodies against the thyroid gland (see 'Causes of hypothyroidism' later in this chapter) develop overt hypothyroidism. The likelihood of progression is less in people with only high TSH levels (3 per cent) or only high levels of antithyroid antibody (2 per cent).[25] On the other hand, men are more likely than women to move from subclinical to overt hypothyroidism.[4] In other words, even if the biochemical readings are reassuring, you should see your doctor if you experience signs or symptoms that might indicate hypothyroidism (see the next section).

Doctors may also suggest testing whether thyroid disease runs in your family or you have another autoimmune disease. Doctors have identified at least 80 distinct autoimmune diseases that together affect 5–8 per cent of the population. Some of these may increase the risk of thyroid disease. For instance, researchers examined 147 children who had atopic dermatitis (allergic eczema). About 1 in 10 of the children showed increased levels of antithyroid antibodies. It seems that abnormal immunity can cause allergies, especially against food, as well as autoimmune reactions. Indeed, the risk of developing thyroid autoimmunity was around four times higher among people with atopic dermatitis than healthy controls.[36]

Symptoms of hypothyroidism

Hypothyroidism is a clinical mimic: several other diseases could cause many of the hallmark symptoms. So unless you develop goitre or have a blood test, hypothyroidism can prove difficult to diagnose based on the classic symptoms of hypothyroidism, which include:

- Cold intolerance (such as wearing jumpers in the summer or turning the central heating off later in the spring and on earlier in the autumn than other people, or setting a temperature that other people find uncomfortably warm)
- Congestive heart failure
- Constipation
- Depression
- Dry, thicker skin
- Fatigue that gradually gets worse over several weeks or months
- Hair loss
- Heavy periods
- Memory loss
- Weight gain (usually several kilograms).

Not everyone with hypothyroidism develops all these symptoms. Indeed, some older people with hypothyroidism do not develop any of the classic symptoms.[16] To complicate matters further, some symptoms – such as weight gain, depression and fatigue – emerge slowly. As a result, you or your doctor might not realize you have a problem for several years. This contributes to distressing cases where hypothyroidism goes unmanaged and undiagnosed, condemning the unfortunate person to potentially avoidable suffering.

Keep a diary

It is important to be proactive in seeking help. You could note your symptoms over a month or two to help your doctor diagnose the problem. You will find a comprehensive list of signs and symptoms in Table 4.1. You should also note what you were doing when the symptoms emerged.

Hypothyroidism and fatigue

Because thyroid hormone controls the activity of almost every cell, hypothyroidism can leave your entire body feeling slow and sluggish and, not surprisingly, fatigue is one of the most common symptoms.

Chapter 11 offers some tips to help you get a good night's sleep. However, fatigue can arise from numerous causes: too many late nights, working too hard or a bug. If the fatigue does not get better after following the tips, getting some early nights or taking

Table 4.1 Typical symptoms of hypothyroidism

Appearance

 Brittle, dry, thinning hair

 Brittle nails

 Dry, scaly, coarse, thickened skin

 Dull facial expression

 Puffy face, bags under the eyes

 'Queen Anne' sign: a thinning or loss of the outer third of the eyebrows

Physical

 Anaemia

 Breathlessness

 Constipation

 Deafness

 Decreased sweating

 Deep, hoarse, croaky voice

 Early puberty

 Exhaustion, fatigue, tiredness

 Heavy, longer or irregular periods

 Muscle aches, weakness and cramps

 Oversensitivity to or increased awareness of cold

 Pins and needles in fingers and hands (carpal tunnel syndrome)

 Poor libido and fertility problems

 Raised blood pressure and cholesterol

 Slow growth and development (children)

 Slow heart rate

 Swelling of feet

 Unexplained or unexpected weight gain

Psychological/neurological

 Depression, low mood, the 'blues'

 Difficulty concentrating – a feeling of 'mental fog'

 Memory problems, especially in older people

 Sleep problems

 Slow thoughts, movements and speech

Source: Adapted from NHS Choices, the British Thyroid Foundation, and Almandoz and Gharib[22]

a holiday, your tiredness may have another cause, including hypothyroidism.

In addition, if you have chronic fatigue syndrome or fibro-myalgia – pain in muscles throughout the body – you might have undiagnosed hypothyroidism.[7] So it's worth asking your doctor to check your thyroid function.

Hypothyroidism and bowel changes

Bowel changes are common in people with thyroid disease – consti-pation with hypothyroidism and diarrhoea with hyperthyroidism. Sometimes a gastroenterologist diagnoses thyroid disease after the patient is referred to a hospital clinic.[7]

Irritable bowel syndrome (IBS) is another very common ailment: about 15 per cent of people in the UK have IBS, the British Society of Gastroenterology notes. IBS can cause considerable – and often underestimated – distress, undermining sexual relation-ships, concentration, social function, physical appearance and self-confidence.[37,38]

However, diagnosing IBS can pose problems. The gut does not change shape. There are no reliable blood or other diagnostic tests. And several ailments can cause gastrointestinal pain, bloating, loose bowels and constipation, including thyroid disease. In add-ition, GPs understandably worry about missing potentially serious diseases such as colorectal cancer.[38] So the British Society of Gastroenterology suggests seeing your doctor if you experience any of the following:

- Changed bowel habit, especially if you are over 40 years of age;
- Passing blood in your stools or from the anus. Although piles (haemorrhoids) cause many cases of anal bleeding, it's always worth checking;
- Unintentional weight loss of more than 2 kg (4 lbs);
- Diarrhoea that wakes you from sleep;
- Fever.

If your IBS does not improve after changing your diet – such as eating more fibre (page 103) – and treatment with drugs, it might be worth asking your doctor to check your thyroid function.

Heart health and hypothyroidism

Unless our hearts pound 'fit to burst' as we try to keep up with our children or grandchildren in the park; unless we suffer the crippling chest pain of angina; unless we end up in casualty after a heart attack, few of us think about the organ that beats in our chest hour after hour, day after day, year after year.

Yet the heart is remarkable. At rest, a healthy heart typically pumps 60–80 times a minute, 86,000 to 115,000 times every day, or around 3 billion times in 80 years, rarely missing a beat, without our once thinking about it. On average, a healthy heart – which is about the size of your fist and weighs approximately 0.3 kg (10 oz) – pumps your 7 litres (12 pints) of blood along 60,000 miles of blood vessels, moving some 10 tons of blood over a day. Incredibly, if you laid your blood vessels end to end they would go around the equator almost two and a half times. Even at rest, a healthy heart pumps approximately 11,000 litres (2,500 gallons) of blood every day – shifting an Olympic swimming pool's worth of blood in about 9 months.

So everyone needs to keep their heart healthy. However, people with hypothyroidism need to be especially careful:

- Hypothyroidism slows the heart. The sluggish heart does not pump blood efficiently. Indeed, hypothyroidism can reduce the volume of blood pumped by between 30 and 50 per cent compared with healthy people.[6] This reduced cardiac output can lead to heart failure because the blood is not propelled powerfully enough to return to the heart.[22]
- Blood pressure increases in about 30 per cent of people with hypothyroidism, partly to ensure tissues receive enough blood as cardiac output falls. The low level of thyroid hormone means that blood vessels contract around the body, which also drives blood pressure up. If you have hypertension, it is especially important to control the amount of salt you eat (page 98)[6] and eat a healthy diet more generally.
- Your liver makes most of the cholesterol in your blood from saturated (animal) fat. Your liver can become sluggish and so levels of 'bad' LDL-cholesterol rise.[7] Around 90 per cent of people with hypothyroidism show dangerously raised levels of cholesterol,[6] which increases the risk of cardiovascular disease.

These changes mean that older people with hypothyroidism may develop angina or intermittent claudication. Angina's crippling chest pain occurs when the heart's demand for oxygen outstrips supply. A reduced blood supply to your legs can cause intermittent claudication (from the Latin for 'to limp'). People with intermittent claudication report aching or cramping pain, with tightness or fatigue in their leg muscles or buttocks. While the pain of intermittent claudication and angina subside after a few minutes' rest, the discomfort may be a warning that you are especially likely to suffer a heart attack. So tell your doctor.

Although hypothyroidism increases cardiovascular risk, treatment usually reverses the problems.[6] Nevertheless, it is especially important to follow a heart-healthy lifestyle, even once your thyroid test has returned to normal. My book *The Heart Attack Survival Guide* contains numerous suggestions for reducing your risk of heart disease.

Blood clots and thyroid disease

Blood clots (coagulation) stop you from bleeding to death from a scratch. However, blood clots inside your body can reduce the amount of blood that reaches an important organ. For example, most heart attacks and many strokes occur when a clot blocks the blood supply to the heart or brain, respectively.

Kate's story

Kate, a 47-year-old office worker, started feeling pins and needles in her hand, her thumb felt weak and her arm ached. At first, she assumed that her workstation was not set up correctly. However, adjusting the layout did not really help.

She also felt tired, with heavy bags under her eyes, could not shake a persistent low mood and the office never felt warm enough, although her colleagues complained that the room was sweltering. Despite sticking to a diet, her weight crept up. When her periods started to be unusually heavy, she started worrying that she might have cancer and saw her GP. Blood tests revealed high TSH and low T_4. Her doctor explained that hypothyroidism might cause nerve damage and trigger carpal tunnel syndrome, which causes pain, numbness and tingling in the hand and fingers as well as dull aches in the arm.

Stroke's sobering statistics

The Stroke Association says that about 152,000 people in the UK suffer a stroke each year – that's about one person every 5 minutes. One in five strokes are fatal. Overall, strokes account for about 1 in 14 deaths in the UK among men and 1 in 10 among women. A stroke leaves half the survivors permanently, and often severely, disabled. People who have had a stroke often experience problems walking, bathing, dressing, eating and going to the lavatory.

Doctors recognize several types of stroke. A build-up of fat in your blood vessels (atherosclerosis) can narrow the arteries that supply the brain with blood. This narrowing reduces or can totally block the flow of blood to the brain, causing 'ischaemic' strokes and transient ischaemic attacks (mini-strokes). Sometimes, a fragment of a clot elsewhere in the body can break off (embolus) and block a vessel supplying the brain, which occurs in some people with an abnormal heartbeat called atrial fibrillation (page 54). In other cases, a blood vessel can rupture and the blood floods into the brain – a 'haemorrhagic' stroke. Whether a clot or a burst vessel causes the stroke, brain cells die within a few minutes – unless the flow of blood restarts rapidly – causing irreversible damage and sometimes permanent disability.

In other words, the body treads a fine line between protecting us from bleeding to death and forming potentially deadly or debilitating clots. The coordinated action of numerous proteins, which form the 'coagulation cascade', is essential to maintain this balance. Indeed, for many biologists the coagulation cascade is one of the most elegant and, in evolutionary terms, remarkable pathways.

Acquired von Willebrand syndrome emerges when you have reduced levels of two proteins (factor VIII and von Willebrand factor) in this coagulation cascade. Doctors refer to the syndrome as 'acquired' because you were not born with the disease, unlike, for example, most cases of haemophilia. Up to about a third of people with recently diagnosed overt hypothyroidism develop acquired von Willebrand syndrome. Symptoms can range from nosebleeds, easy bruising or excessive blood loss after dental procedures to, in rare cases, major loss of blood, especially following an operation or accident. Fortunately, the bleeding problems linked to hypothyroidism usually improve after treatment.[39] So if you find you bleed or bruise easily, see your doctor.

Causes of hypothyroidism

Worldwide, iodine deficiency is the most common cause of hypothyroidism. However, in parts of the world where doctors believe that there is sufficient iodine in the diet, about 1 person in every 200 still develops hypothyroidism.[1] Clearly, iodine deficiency is not the only cause.

In the rest of the world, treatments for hyperthyroidism (see Chapter 5) that destroy part of the thyroid gland cause up to one-third of cases of hypothyroidism.[25] Indeed, sometimes surgeons deliberately cause hypothyroidism to make sure the gland no longer works. This may reduce the risk of, for example, cancer recurrence. In addition, between 10 and 45 per cent of people treated with radiotherapy for head and neck cancer develop hypothyroidism.[22] The British Thyroid Foundation notes that doctors in the UK do not usually use radiotherapy for head and neck cancer, although the approach is more common in some other countries.

Autoantibodies against the thyroid seem to cause most of the remaining cases of hypothyroidism, as we'll see later in the chapter. However, numerous other factors can lower levels of thyroid hormone:

- Thyroid function declines with age as the gland wastes away – a change called spontaneous atrophic hypothyroidism.[7]
- Pregnancy (Chapter 8).
- Developmental problems in the womb. Around 1 child in every 3,500 is born with congenital hypothyroidism (page 88).
- Some supplements, such as kelp, can trigger hypothyroidism if taken in large doses (page 96). Other supplements (such as iron and calcium) can reduce the amount of levothyroxine you absorb,[22] tipping you into hypothyroidism. So always check with your doctor before using supplements if you have or are at risk of hypothyroidism, for example if your TSH levels are raised or you have a family history of thyroid disease.
- Diseases affecting the pituitary gland can compromise thyroid function. As mentioned in Chapter 1, the pituitary is a master gland that controls the thyroid.
- Some infections (page 92) may damage the thyroid gland, at least temporarily.
- Numerous medicines can trigger hypothyroidism or make

matters worse if you have an underactive thyroid (page 90). In some cases, these may tip the balance into overt hypothyroidism. Always remind your doctor and let your pharmacist know if you have hypothyroidism, informing them of any other drugs you are taking, even when buying a medicine without a prescription.

Hashimoto's thyroiditis

Hakaru Hashimoto, a Japanese surgeon, described the thyroiditis that now bears his name in 1912. Hashimoto's is a type of autoimmune thyroiditis, which arises when the immune system mistakenly attacks thyroid cells.

Antibodies against the thyroid are remarkably common. Indeed, up to a fifth of otherwise healthy women show mild autoimmune thyroiditis, according to the British Thyroid Foundation. Men are between four and ten times less likely to develop thyroiditis than women. However, showing antibodies on a blood test does not inevitably mean that you will develop symptoms. The British Thyroid Foundation remarks that only about 10 per cent of people with autoimmune thyroiditis develop symptoms of hypothyroidism or goitre.[25] So how does this common disease develop?

Protecting us from harm

Threats to our health and well-being, such as viruses, bacteria, parasites and fungi, are all around us. According to Bill Bryson, your skin is home to around a trillion bacteria – that's 100,000 on each centimetre – although not all these are harmful. Our immune system protects us from dangerous pathogens, and antibodies are one of the most important lines of immune defence.

Antibodies are Y-shaped proteins produced by certain white blood cells. Antibodies 'tag' an invading microbe or an infected cell. These tags allow other white blood cells to home in on and destroy the invader or damaged cell. Antibodies may also directly attack microbes by, for example, blocking part of a bacterium essential for its survival.

Antibodies are exquisitely specific: they recognize, for example, only a tiny area of a particular protein on a certain bacterium. Scientists call this target the 'antigen'. Your body produces antibodies against some 100 million different antigens. This vast repertoire protects you from the thousands of potential threats you encounter every day.

Normally, however, the cells of your body do not trigger antibody production; the immune system recognizes that they belong to the body it is trying to protect. Sometimes, however, things go wrong: an antibody mistakes normal, healthy cells for 'invaders'. So the antibody 'tags' the normal cell. In response, white blood cells attack and destroy the healthy tissue. Once the damage exceeds the body's ability to compensate, the person develops signs and symptoms of an autoimmune disease. For example:

- People develop rheumatoid arthritis after the immune system attacks the joints.
- Multiple sclerosis follows an immune attack on the fatty myelin sheath that surrounds many nerves. This reduces the nerve's ability to conduct signals.
- If antibodies destroy insulin-producing cells in the pancreas, a person may develop type 1 diabetes.
- If the body mistakenly attacks the outer layer (cortex) of the adrenal glands, a person may develop Addison's disease. The adrenal glands lie on top of the kidneys. The adrenal cortex releases two hormones that help control blood pressure – cortisol and aldosterone.

In Hashimoto's thyroiditis, white blood cells invade the gland and secrete antibodies that target and inactivate thyroid peroxidase (page 16). Over many years, the white blood cells destroy the thyroid gland. However, the attack waxes and wanes. From time to time the disease may seem to lie dormant. Nevertheless, the auto-immune attack eventually flares.[4]

Doctors look for antibodies against thyroid peroxidase (also called thyroperoxidase) in a blood sample to help diagnose Hashimoto's thyroiditis. Levels of the antibodies tend to rise as Hashimoto's thyroiditis progresses. However, if the autoimmune attack totally destroys the gland, the levels of the antibody may be very low or even undetectable.[4]

The symptoms of Hashimoto's thyroiditis may vary over time. For example, the first sign may be a small, painless or slightly uncomfortable goitre. Other people experience mild hyperthyroidism for a few weeks or months – a phenomenon called hashitoxicosis. The symptoms are often similar to Graves' disease and can include eye changes (Chapters 5 and 6). These symptoms arise because the antibodies initially stimulate the gland before the destruction causes hypothyroidism. Eventually, however, people with Hashimoto's thyroiditis develop the signs and symptoms of hypothyroidism.[4]

Scientists do not really understand why the immune system loses tolerance to, and starts attacking, the thyroid gland or other tissues. However, it's clear that people with some other autoimmune diseases are at markedly increased risk of producing antibodies against thyroid peroxidase, including 20–30 per cent of those with type 1 diabetes and around 80 per cent of those with Addison's disease.[4]

Treating hypothyroidism

Victorian patients with hypothyroidism ate fried, minced thyroid gland served on bread to give them a boost. Then, in 1891, the British physicians Victor Horsley and George Murray began treating hypothyroidism with extracts of thyroid gland.[21] By the middle of the twentieth century, doctors had started using dried extract of thyroid gland. However, because the drug came from animals, no two preparations were exactly the same.[7]

Today, doctors use a synthetic, standardized version of the hormone called levothyroxine to replace missing T_4. The number of prescriptions for levothyroxine in the UK increased from 7 million in 1998 to 23.4 million in 2010. This increase partly reflects a tendency to prescribe levothyroxine for more marginal – in other words, subclinical – hypothyroidism.[5]

It is essential to follow your doctor's instructions to avoid triggering overactivity in your thyroid while alleviating the symptoms of hypothyroidism. If you do not take enough levothyroxine, symptoms may re-emerge and your doctor will not know whether the recurrence represents a worsening of the disease or whether the symptoms reflect your poor adherence to your treatment – in other words, how well you follow your doctor's advice. On the other hand, being slightly thyrotoxic can give a feeling of being 'high' and some people take too much 'in the mistaken hope' that they will lose weight more rapidly.[4]

The British Thyroid Foundation notes that levothyroxine has 'negligible' side effects. But taking excessive amounts can leave you at risk of heart problems and osteoporosis.[4] So you need to discuss the risks and benefits of treatment with your doctor. If you are still worried, ask for a referral to a specialist. After all, a GP cannot be an expert in everything.

> ### Helping adherence
>
> Partners, family members and other carers can improve your adherence by helping you establish a routine for taking levothyroxine and other medicines. Some partners and family members write a list of the medicines to be taken and when. You could give this list to an unfamiliar doctor (such as when you are on holiday), to accident and emergency staff and to pharmacists if you are buying medication. Some medicines can interact with another drug and even supplements or medicines bought without a prescription, either causing side effects or undermining the effectiveness of one drug or the other. These interactions pose a particular problem for people taking levothyroxine, as we will discuss later in the chapter.

You will probably take levothyroxine for the rest of your life. Occasionally, however, people may be able to stop treatment. Older people, in particular, may still take levothyroxine after transient hypothyroidism resolves or after a misdiagnosis many years ago when doctors understood less about thyroid disease. In one study, doctors safely stopped levothyroxine in half of those taking the treatment in a nursing home.[16] However, never stop or reduce the dose of any treatment without speaking to your doctor first.

Why not use T_3?

The body breaks T_3 down rapidly, much more quickly than T_4. So you would need to take T_3 several times a day and levels of the thyroid hormone and TSH would fluctuate widely. As a result, doctors generally do not use T_3 alone.[22] However, they may suggest T_3 before giving radioiodine to treat or scan for thyroid cancer. They may also use T_3 in the unlikely event you suffer a myxoedema coma.[4]

Some doctors may suggest adding T_3 if you still experience marked fatigue, weight problems, and poor mood and thinking while taking levothyroxine alone.[22] However, some studies suggest that the combination is no more effective than levothyroxine alone. And some trials suggest that symptoms worsen in patients who also receive T_3. Future formulations that release T_3 slowly over several hours may change the balance of risks and benefits.[4]

In the meantime, one of the problems of clinical studies is that they average the results from a large number of people. Therefore, just because a treatment does not work in 'the average patient', that does not necessarily mean it will not work in you. As we have seen, the reference ranges used for thyroid disease are based on the general population, not personalized to you. So if you want to try a course of T_3, feel free to ask to discuss the risks and benefits with a specialist. I would suggest keeping a diary to track the benefits and possible side effects of T_3 and, indeed, any treatment.

Getting the most from levothyroxine

The British Thyroid Foundation says that most people with hypo-thyroidism need between 125 and 150 micrograms of levothyroxine each day. (A microgram [μg] is a millionth of a gram and is some-times also written as 'mcg'.) Your doctor will tailor the treatment to your needs and, occasionally, the dose is as little as 25 μg or as much as 200 μg.[4]

You should take levothyroxine on an empty stomach at the same time each day, and ideally 1 hour before breakfast and at least 4 hours after your last meal. Taking levothyroxine regularly and well before eating any food that could interfere with absorption helps tightly control TSH. Your doctor will also advise you not to eat or drink for 30 minutes to 1 hour afterwards.[24] You should ask your doctor what to do if you miss a dose.

Food, as well as certain supplements and medicines, can interfere with the absorption of levothyroxine. So do not take other supple-ments or medicines for at least 1 hour after taking levothyroxine.[22] The British Thyroid Foundation suggests avoiding calcium, iron, some cholesterol-lowering drugs and multivitamins for at least 4 hours before and after levothyroxine. On the other hand, grape-fruit juice seems to increase the amount of levothyroxine you absorb – so it is probably best avoided. If you are unsure, speak to your doctor or pharmacist.

Diseases that can reduce levothyroxine absorption

Some diseases can reduce the amount of levothyroxine you absorb.[24] These include:

- Coeliac disease: a gastrointestinal reaction to gluten, the mix of two proteins in wheat, barley and rye that gives dough its elasticity.
- Infection with a bacterium called *Helicobacter pylori*. Remarkably, *H. pylori* thrives in the strong acid in your stomach and can cause ulcers and stomach cancer. *H. pylori* may also reduce acid secretion, which can change the amount of levothyroxine you absorb.
- Autoimmune gastritis, which also reduces acid secretion.

Your doctor should know from your records whether you have one of these conditions. However, mention any other disease you have to your doctor and pharmacist, just to be on the safe side.

Tailoring treatment

The amount of levothyroxine needed varies from person to person. Your doctor will carefully adjust the dose to ensure you do not develop hypothyroidism, while avoiding problems linked to excessive levels. This means that you will need blood tests once every 6–8 weeks or so until your thyroid function tests return to normal. You will usually then have a test every year, although the frequency depends on your individual circumstances. However, always see your doctor if symptoms of hyperthyroidism or hypothyroidism emerge between your scheduled blood tests.

Your doctor may increase the dose more gradually if you have severe hypothyroidism or you have another ailment, especially heart disease. Thyroid hormone increases the amount of oxygen used by the heart. As a result, high levels of thyroid hormone can trigger angina attacks, abnormal heartbeats and even heart attacks. Older people, especially those with heart disease, seem to be the most vulnerable to these effects. If you experience more frequent or severe angina attacks, difficulty breathing, confusion, insomnia or any new or changed symptom, see your doctor as soon as possible. It's also worth making sure that your spouse, children and other caregivers know the warning signs.[16] You could, for example, keep a diary in which you note any symptoms, their severity and possible triggers.

But you will need to be patient: the British Thyroid Foundation points out that you may need to take levothyroxine for several months before you feel back to normal. As the improvement is gradual, keeping a diary can help you see how far you have come. Furthermore, some people do not feel completely well despite having normal TSH levels. So let your doctor know: altering the levothyroxine dosage to bring TSH levels into the lower half of the normal range may help.[24] As always, never change the dose of a drug without speaking to your doctor first. Indeed, suppressing TSH to below the lower limit of the normal range may increase the risk of atrial fibrillation (page 54), which is linked to stroke, and osteoporosis.[24]

Finally, if you want to have a baby or have an unplanned pregnancy, see your doctor as soon as possible (see Chapter 8). And because many thyroid diseases run in families, it is worth your relatives discussing with their doctors whether to have their thyroid function tested.

5

Hyperthyroidism

Hyperthyroidism – increased production of thyroid hormone – is also relatively common. And, once again, women are particularly likely to develop hyperthyroidism. In areas of the world where doctors consider that iodine intakes are adequate, about 1 in 50 women and 1 in 500 men develop thyrotoxicosis (page 6).[1] In addition, between 1 in 160 and 1 in 50 people develop subclinical hyperthyroidism.[26] Graves' disease accounts for more than four-fifths of these cases. However, toxic nodular goitre (page 19) becomes an increasingly important cause of subclinical hyperthyroidism among older people.[4,25]

Graves' disease

In 1825, a posthumous collection of writings by Caleb Parry, a doctor from Bath (then a popular health resort), described the case of 21-year-old Elizabeth S, who fell from a wheelchair while moving down a hill. Although not badly hurt, she was terrified. Shortly after, Elizabeth felt nervous, suffered palpitations and her thyroid swelled.[40] Parry had described the ailment we now call Graves' disease. Elizabeth's case highlights the intimate relationship between emotions, stress and thyroid disease, an issue we will return to in Chapter 11.[18]

Despite Parry's observations, the illness is named after Robert Graves, a doctor working in Dublin, who described a patient with goitre and thyroid eye disease (Chapter 6) in 1835. In mainland Europe, doctors sometimes call the condition von Basedow's disease, after Carl von Basedow, who described the ailment in 1840.[4]

Until modern treatments, the disease was, indeed, grave. About 20 per cent of people with Graves' disease died from the illness. The rest suffered years of ill health characterized by relapses and remissions.[4] Today, most people with Graves' disease live full and fulfilled lives, although symptoms tend to improve slowly once treatment begins.[24]

The elusive cause of Graves' disease

The cause of Graves' disease remained a mystery for more than a century after the early descriptions. Parry and Graves blamed heart disease: Graves' disease can cause pulmonary hypertension (dangerously raised blood pressure in the lung), which can end in heart failure (page 31). Graves' disease also increases the risk of death from cardiovascular causes.[6] Other doctors, because of the marked tremor experienced by many patients, blamed a nervous ailment.[6] Hormones also contribute: as mentioned at the start of the chapter, women are around ten times more likely than men to develop Graves' disease.[4]

Over the years, however, researchers identified abnormalities in the thyroid as the source of Graves' disease. In 1956, scientists discovered a protein in the blood of people with Graves' disease that they called 'long-acting thyroid stimulator' (LATS). In animals, LATS stimulated the gland for longer than TSH.[7] In 1978, researchers discovered that LATS was an antibody that bound to and stimulated the TSH receptor (page 9).[40] In other words, Graves' disease is another example of an autoimmune disease (page 40). Instead of attacking an invading microbe, autoantibodies mistakenly stimulate the receptor, tricking the gland into responding as it would when TSH binds, although the effect is much longer lasting.[41]

Researchers now believe that an environmental factor – such as increased iodine consumption, stress or a viral infection – triggers Graves' disease in genetically susceptible people.[4] Indeed, the spouse of a person with Graves' disease is almost three times more likely than the general population to develop the disorder,[42] which indicates that part of the risk is environmental.

Nevertheless, genes (page 00) seem to account for about 70–80 per cent of the risk of developing Graves' disease. For example, if one of your brothers or sisters has Graves' disease you are about five times more likely to develop the condition. Having two or more affected siblings increases the risk 310 times![18,40]

The autoimmune family

Furthermore, many people with Graves' disease or members of their family have other autoimmune disorders, such as:

- Pernicious anaemia: your body cannot absorb vitamin B_{12}. Your red blood cells need B_{12} to work properly, and the deficiency arising from the poor absorption means you develop anaemia.
- Vitiligo: areas of skin depigmentation.
- Addison's disease (page 41).
- Coeliac disease (page 45).
- Type 1 diabetes: the type that generally emerges in childhood.[24] NHS Choices notes that hyperthyroidism can exacerbate the symptoms of diabetes, including thirst and tiredness.

It seems that some people inherit a tendency to mount autoimmune attacks, which can emerge in a variety of ways, depending on the environmental trigger and the rest of their genetic background.

Symptoms and signs of hyperthyroidism

Exophthalmos – staring, bulging eyes (Chapter 6) – is probably the most striking, distressing and well-known manifestation of thyrotoxicosis.[4] However, as Table 5.1 shows, hyperthyroidism can cause numerous other problems.

Not everyone with hyperthyroidism develops all these symptoms, and the speed of onset differs. Typically, thyrotoxicosis develops gradually over several months. Occasionally, however, the signs and symptoms emerge in a few days or weeks.[4] Moreover some people, especially those with Graves' disease, swing from no symptoms to thyrotoxicosis and then to hypothyroidism and back to hyperthyroidism. Eventually, about 1 in 20 people with Graves' disease develop persistent hypothyroidism: they become passive, lethargic and may even remain in bed all day.[7] Given the variable course, the wide range of symptoms and the considerable overlap with other diseases, it is worth keeping a diary, noting when and where your symptoms occur (page 12).

Table 5.1 Typical symptoms of hyperthyroidism

Appearance

Loss of nails

Patchy hair loss

Red palms

Slightly reddened, raised and thickened patches of skin on the lower part of the leg, which may spread to the foot; hair in this area can become coarser

'Staring', 'startled' appearance

Physical

Children may be clumsy and tall for their age

Excessive sweating (e.g. warm, moist palms and skin)

Feeling tired all the time

Frequently passing stools or urine or both

Goitre – although the size of the gland may be normal

Greasy, 'fatty' stools

Heat intolerance (e.g. wearing light clothing even in cold weather)

Increased appetite

Infrequent, light or no periods

Infertility and lack of interest in sex

Itchy skin, but not a rash

Muscle weakness and twitches in the face and limbs

Rapid or irregular heartbeat or both, even when asleep

Tremor, trembling, shaking, restlessness

Unexplained or unexpected weight loss

Psychological/neurological

Anxiety

Irritability

Nervousness

Hyperactivity

Sleep problems

Source: Adapted from NHS Choices and Vanderpump and Tunbridge[4]

Abigail's story

Abigail – a 50-year-old mother of three, who works part-time at her local supermarket – recently saw her GP as she felt constantly on edge, tired all the time and just could not sit still. 'She's on a short fuse', Abigail's husband told friends. Abigail also felt hot and sweaty at work and she had asked her manager several times whether the heating was too high. Her colleagues wondered how she could go into the cold store without wearing a cardigan.

Abigail also found stacking increasing difficult, especially the higher and lower shelves, and felt increasingly breathless carrying bags back from the shops or climbing stairs. Yet she was losing weight. 'And a good thing too,' she told the doctor, 'but I can't understand why I don't feel fitter.'

'My mother died six months back, but I've got nothing much to worry about', she told the doctor. Abigail also kept kicking the duvet off at night, which her husband blamed on hot flushes. Abigail wondered whether her husband was right. However, her daughter had read about thyroid disease and suggested thyroid function tests. These revealed hyperthyroidism.

As Abigail found, tiredness is a common early symptom of hyperthyroidism and may gradually worsen as the illness develops. In other cases, staring – caused as the upper lids pull back away from the eyeball – is the first hint (Chapter 6). Hyperthyroidism's other common signs and symptoms include:[4,26]

- Palpitations: increased awareness of the heartbeat
- Nervousness and irritability
- Tremor, which can be marked
- Sweating
- Loose bowels, an urgent need to defecate and, in some cases, diarrhoea
- Heat intolerance: feeling excessively hot, almost as if the heating is too high
- Poor concentration, mood swings and altered perception
- Behaviour changes: people with hyperthyroidism may talk a lot, pace up and down, and seem almost manic
- Breathlessness on exercise
- Feeling weak, which affects men in particular and is especially common in the upper muscles of the arms and legs

- Increased appetite or feeling hungry all the time, and despite losing weight.

The pattern of symptoms can change as you get older. For example, some older people with hyperthyroidism do not develop the 'hyperdynamic' symptoms that are common in younger people, such as tremor, intolerance to heat, eye changes, nervousness and fast heartbeat. These hyperdynamic symptoms are especially unlikely to emerge if their hyperthyroidism has not been treated for several years. Instead, older people may seem lethargic, almost sedated, apathetic and depressed. They may eat poorly but still seem bloated. The gland tends not to be enlarged and eye disease is unusual. Even the pulse may be slow or normal.[4] Not surprisingly, doctors may miss or misdiagnose (for instance, as depression), this 'apathetic hyperthyroidism'.

Thyroid storms

Occasionally, thyrotoxicosis triggers a sudden and severe exacerbation of the hyperthyroid symptoms, called a thyroid storm. Several factors, including infections, injury or surgery, and not taking medicines as recommended, can trigger a thyroid storm in susceptible people.[18] Usually, however, thyroid storms follow another illness, such as pneumonia, stress or a psychiatric disturbance, or treatment with radioiodine.[4]

The hormonal tsunami released during a thyroid storm can cause a fever; rapid heartbeat or atrial fibrillation; heart failure; profound sweating (which can result in dehydration); vomiting; diarrhoea; confusion; shock and delirium. Untreated, the patient may slip into a coma or even die. So you should go to accident and emergency if your symptoms suddenly worsen.[4,18] Thankfully, thyroid storms are relatively rare.

Hyperthyroidism and the heart

Thyroid hormone increases the amount of energy that almost every organ burns. For instance, the heart may beat excessively. Indeed, cardiovascular symptoms are often the main consequence of hyperthyroidism in people with Graves' disease who are over 55 years of age.

The heart's four chambers – two atria and two ventricles – beat in sequence, pushing that 10 tons of blood around your body

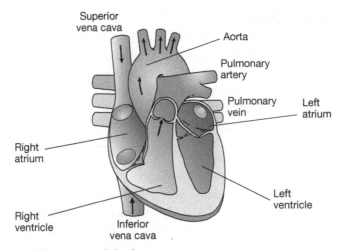

Figure 5.1 Structure of the heart

every day. The atria collect blood from the circulation. When they contract, the atria push blood into the ventricles. The two atria are smaller and weaker than the ventricles, which push blood around thousands of miles of blood vessels. The right atrium and right ventricle pump blood to the lungs. The left atrium and left ventricle pump blood around the rest of the body. That's why the left ventricle is much more muscular than the right ventricle (Figure 5.1).

So people with Graves' disease and other forms of hyperthyroidism might experience a number of symptoms that might be linked to heart disease, including:[4,6]

- Shortness of breath: especially lying down, which can make sleeping difficult (see page 113 for some tips on sleeping well).
- Swollen ankles: which might indicate heart failure (page 31).
- Atrial fibrillation (next page): if you have an irregular heartbeat or palpitations, it is worth asking your doctor to check your pulse and, if it is abnormal, to perform a thyroid function test.
- Increased cardiac output: the volume of blood pumped by the heart can increase by 50–300 per cent in hyperthyroidism.
- Hypertension: if you have high blood pressure it is worth asking your doctor to check your thyroid function.

What is atrial fibrillation?

Between 2 and 15 per cent of people with hyperthyroidism develop an abnormal heartbeat called atrial fibrillation, and the risk seems to rise with advancing age.[6] Atrial fibrillation increases the risk of stroke between four- and fivefold, doubles the risk of dementia and triples the risk of heart failure.[43] Atrial fibrillation is three times more common in people with low TSH levels than in those with normal concentrations.[4] So what is atrial fibrillation? And why is it so dangerous?

Arrhythmias are changes in the heart's rate or rhythm. The heart may beat too quickly (tachycardia), too slowly (bradycardia) or irregularly. Most arrhythmias are harmless, but some are serious or even life-threatening. In atrial fibrillation, the atria beat up to 400 times per minute. This means that the heart only has the time to partially contract. Furthermore, the contractions of the atria and ventricles are uncoordinated: the ventricles contract between 140 and 180 times a minute and the force of the contractions varies considerably. As a result, atrial fibrillation can cut the amount of blood pumped by the heart by 15–20 per cent.[44] Because the heart pumps less effectively, people with atrial fibrillation experience breathlessness (often the first symptom), palpitations and dizziness.

In addition, the uncoordinated contractions can leave blood behind in the heart's chambers. And this blood can clot, which is potentially dangerous (page 37). For instance, fragments of these clots can break away and lodge in the small vessels supplying the brain. Indeed, atrial fibrillation may underlie up to a quarter of strokes.[43]

So ask your doctor or nurse to measure your pulse. Everyone who has an irregular pulse should have an ECG, whether or not you experience symptoms. Likewise, doctors should check thyroid hormone and TSH levels in any person with atrial fibrillation.

Subclinical hyperthyroidism

People with subclinical hyperthyroidism show low levels of TSH and normal levels of T_3 and T_4 – a pattern that can arise from numerous causes. About half of people with subclinical hyperthyroidism take levothyroxine to treat hypothyroidism. So if you develop symptoms of hyperthyroidism, you might want to discuss reducing your dose of levothyroxine with your doctor. However, never change the dose or stop taking a treatment without speaking to your doctor first.

Several other ailments can underlie subclinical hyperthyroidism, including:[25]

- a mildly overactive thyroid gland;
- certain diseases of the hypothalamus or pituitary;
- some illnesses affecting organs other than the thyroid;
- taking drugs that reduce TSH secretion.

Symptoms of subclinical hyperthyroidism

Fortunately, relatively few people with subclinical hyperthyroidism eventually develop thyrotoxicosis. In one study, just 0.5–0.7 per cent of people with at least two low serum TSH measurements developed hyperthyroidism during follow-up lasting between 4 months and 7 years.[25] The risk increases with age: about 1–2 per cent of people aged over 60 who have subclinical hyperthyroidism develop the full-blown disease.[26] Nevertheless, subclinical hyperthyroidism can cause symptoms:

- Osteoporosis (page 6): subclinical hyperthyroidism does not seem to increase fracture risk in either premenopausal women or men. However, it can decrease bone mass and accelerate osteoporosis in postmenopausal women, who are already vulnerable to brittle bone disease. In one study, women aged 65 years or older who had low TSH levels were four times more likely to have vertebral (spinal) fractures and three times more likely to break their hips than those with levels in the normal range.[25] So it's important to ensure you get enough calcium and vitamin D.[16]
- Atrial fibrillation:[26] people with subclinical hyperthyroidism often have increased heart rate and are at increased risk of atrial and ventricular arrhythmias. For example, 10–13 per cent of elderly people with subclinical hyperthyroidism develop atrial fibrillation, compared with 2–5 per cent of those with normal thyroid function.[25] Some studies suggest that subclinical hyperthyroidism might carry the same increased risk of atrial fibrillation as the full-blown disease.[6]
- People with subclinical hyperthyroidism are just over twice as

likely to show poor memory and mental abilities as those with a normally functioning thyroid.[16]

Despite the growing recognition that subclinical hyperthyroidism causes symptoms, doctors are not sure how best to manage the disease, or even whether to treat it at all.[8] Some doctors advocate treating subclinical hyperthyroidism to prevent atrial fibrillation, osteoporotic fractures and overt hyperthyroidism – and, they suggest, save lives.[25] However, not every doctor agrees and all treatments have risks. So it is important to have a full and frank discussion with your doctor.

Treating hyperthyroidism

Provided you take your medicines as prescribed by your doctor, drugs control about 90 per cent of cases of hyperthyroidism.[18] Nevertheless, hyperthyroidism often recurs if you stop taking treatment. About two-thirds of relapses occur during the year after treatment stops. Relapses more than 10 years after the end of treatment with antithyroid drugs are unusual. People with large goitres, those with severe hyperthyroidism and those with a high dietary iodine intake (such as from seaweed or kelp tablets) are the most likely to relapse, which might need treatment with radioiodine or surgery.[24] On the other hand, between 5 and 20 per cent of people treated with antithyroid drugs develop hypothyroidism, sometimes up to 10–15 years after the overactivity settles. This seems to be due to autoimmune damage.[4,24]

Antithyroid drugs

Carbimazole is the most widely used antithyroid drug in the UK. However, your doctor may suggest propylthiouracil if you develop side effects while taking carbimazole. Furthermore, propylthiouracil, unlike carbimazole, reduces the conversion of T_4 to T_3. This additional action makes propylthiouracil useful for severe thyrotoxicosis, including a 'storm'. However, you may need to take up to 9 or even 12 propylthiouracil tablets each day.[24]

Titration regimen

Doctors will adjust the dose of the antithyroid drug to ensure that you get the most benefit, while minimizing side effects. For example, doctors may give 20 mg of carbimazole two or three times daily (or the equivalent dose of propylthiouracil) and reduce the dose every 3–6 weeks, based on free T_4 measurements, to achieve a maintenance daily dose (typically 5–10 mg). Titration may take between 18 and 24 months.[24] Using the lowest effective dose of antithyroid drug allows doctors to judge the aggressiveness of the underlying thyroid disease. Doctors also titrate treatment for women who are breastfeeding or pregnant.[4]

Block regimen

Alternatively, doctors may prescribe carbimazole at 20 mg two or three times daily (or the equivalent of propylthiouracil) and after about 4 weeks add levothyroxine. Doctors will also adjust the levo-thyroxine dose based on free T_4 levels. The dose of the antithyroid drug remains constant. Titration may take about 6 months.[24] This 'block' regimen avoids swings between over- and underactivity that can emerge if the dose needs regular adjustment during the titration regimen. Moreover, antithyroid drugs may suppress the autoimmune attack on the gland, so some specialists use a block regimen to treat severe active eye disease.[4]

Side effects of antithyroid drugs

Side effects from antithyroid drugs are most common during the first 3 months of treatment, when the patient takes high doses. Between 2 and 5 per cent of those taking an antithyroid drug develop relatively minor side effects, including:[4,24]

- Pruritus (itching)
- Arthralgia (joint pains)
- Fever
- Gastrointestinal upset (usually mild)
- Altered taste
- Rash (in 5–10 per cent of people).

Serious side effects are less common, occurring in fewer than 1 in 500 patients. See your doctor if you develop symptoms that might indicate liver damage, such as pain in the upper abdomen, unexpected weight loss and widespread itching. Furthermore, each year about 3 in every 10,000 people taking antithyroid drugs show a dangerous decline in their level of neutrophils – a type of white blood cell. Doctors call this agranulocytosis. Why antithyroid drugs reduce levels of these disease-fighting cells remains a mystery.[4] However, carbimazole has caused fatal agranulocytosis – although try to keep the risks in perspective. Agranulocytosis is very rare.

Watch for the warning signs of agranulocytosis

Nevertheless, you need to watch for signs of an infection. Your doctor will tell you when to stop your tablets and you may need antibiotics until your bone marrow – which makes white blood cells – recovers.[4] Your doctor may tell you, if you suffer sore throats, bruising or bleeding, mouth ulcers, fever or feel generally unwell, to stop taking the tablets and seek medical help immediately. As agranulocytosis can be fatal, it is important that you, your partner and family know the warning signs and what to do.

Other drugs for hyperthyroidism

Doctors may suggest one or more other drugs, depending on your particular problem. For example, hyperthyroidism can trigger anxiety, a racing heart, tremor and muscular weakness. Beta-blockers block the receptor for adrenaline (page 9) and so can control hyperactivity of the heart, sweating, anxiety and restless-ness. Beta-blockers are not cures, but can make you feel more comfortable. While they are generally safe, you must let your doctor know if you have asthma because beta-blockers sometimes trigger asthma attacks in susceptible people.[4]

Several other drugs might help in certain circumstances:

- Your doctor may suggest prednisolone, a type of steroid, to reduce inflammation caused by severe subacute thyroiditis (page 93). Once the inflammation is controlled, you will gradually reduce the dose of steroid over 2–4 weeks.[24]
- Painkillers (analgesics), including paracetamol, usually resolve mild thyroid tenderness.[24]
- Occasionally, conventional antithyroid drugs fail or their side effects mean you cannot take them. In these cases, potassium perchlorate or lithium can reduce thyroid hormone production. But both have serious side effects.[24]
- Potassium perchlorate is sometimes used for hyperthyroidism caused by excessive iodine intake, including thyrotoxicosis caused by amiodarone (page 90).[24]

- Atrial fibrillation caused by hyperthyroidism resolves in about half of patients when the overactivity of the gland normalizes. If not, you may need warfarin and digoxin, which prevent clots and help establish a normal rhythm, respectively.[24] In a recent UK study, warfarin halved the risk of stroke in people with atrial fibrillation.[45]

Radiotherapy

Doctors have used radioiodine to treat Graves' disease for more than 60 years.[4] Radioiodine destroys active areas ('hot') of the thyroid gland (page 19), which brings levels of thyroid hormone back to within the normal range. A single dose of radioiodine successfully treats about 90 per cent of people with Graves' disease, [24] with the benefits usually emerging between 6 weeks and 3 months after treatment.[18] Most of the remainder respond to a second dose, usually given 6 months later.[24]

Doctors tend to use radioiodine and, less commonly, surgery if hyperthyroidism relapses, rather than as a first-line treatment. Some hospitals, however, recommend radioiodine as the initial treatment, especially if the person is older, has cardiovascular (heart and blood vessel) disease or both.[24] Furthermore, some mothers find looking after a baby difficult while juggling the need for treatment for Graves' disease. As a result, they undergo radiotherapy or surgery before becoming pregnant.[4] You need to discuss the risks and benefits of each approach with your doctor.

Nevertheless, radioiodine has several limitations:

- About 1 per cent of patients experience inflammation soon after receiving radioiodine. So the gland can be tender for a few days.[4,7] However, nausea or significant neck swelling are rare.[18]
- Between 10 and 50 per cent of people with Graves' disease develop hypothyroidism in the first year after receiving radio-iodine. This rises to more than 80 per cent after 20 years.[4,24] These people usually need thyroid replacement therapy for the rest of their lives.[22]
- Radioiodine can exacerbate active eye disease,[4] especially in smokers. So you may need to take prednisolone for 3 months after receiving radioiodine.[24]
- Your doctor may suggest avoiding close and prolonged contact

with other people – especially children and pregnant women – for several weeks after receiving radioiodine.[4] Always make sure you understand any restrictions.

- Most people with Graves' disease take antithyroid drugs before radioiodine to prevent a thyroid storm. As the radioiodine destroys the cells, the stores of thyroid hormones flood into the bloodstream.[7] Nevertheless, thyroid hormone levels may still increase temporarily about 4–10 days after treatment. So your doctor may suggest you take beta-blockers, painkillers or both.

Surgery

You might want to consider surgery if you really want to avoid radioiodine (after a full discussion of the risks and benefits with your doctor), you cannot avoid close contact with children or need rapid removal of a goitre that is cosmetically unsightly or causes breathing difficulties or other problems. Often, surgery aims to remove sufficient gland to cause hypothyroidism. This reduces the likelihood that the hyperthyroidism will recur. However, you will need to take levothyroxine (page 42).[4]

There are several risks associated with surgery, including damage to the parathyroid glands or the nerves supplying the vocal cords. Indeed, the operation can bruise the nerves, leaving your voice hoarse or husky for a few days. The anaesthetic can also temporarily change the tone and character of your voice. Your voice will change permanently only if the surgeon accidently cuts the nerves, but this is rare if the surgeon is experienced.[4]

6

Thyroid eye disease

Apart from goitres, changes to the eyes are generally the most noticeable and characteristic sign of thyroid disease – Patsy Westcott calls the hallmark changes to the eyes 'one of the most cruel and puzzling conditions associated with thyroid disorders'.[7]

Sight is essential for navigating around daily life. Eye contact aids effective communication. And the eyes can be one of the most attractive parts of the body. Understandably therefore, thyroid eye disease (also called thyroid orbitopathy) can dramatically undermine feelings of attractiveness, confidence and self-esteem. In addition, thyroid eye disease occasionally causes blindness from pressure on the optic nerve (which carries messages from the light-sensitive retina that lines the back of the eye to the brain) or ulcers on the cornea, which can interfere with sight (Figure 6.1).

Fewer than 1 in 20 people with thyroid orbitopathy develop 'very severe' eye disease, the British Thyroid Foundation says. Nevertheless, the Royal College of Ophthalmologists estimates that about 400,000 people in the UK have thyroid eye disease – that's more than the population of Coventry. So what can you do?

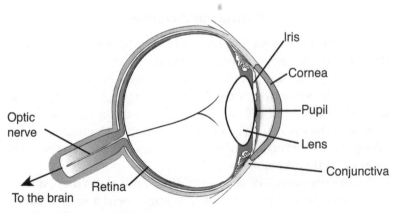

Figure 6.1 Structure of the eye

Causes of orbitopathy

The British Thyroid Foundation notes that Graves' disease (page 47) causes most cases of thyroid eye disease in the UK. Indeed, between a third and a half of people who have Graves' disease develop orbitopathy, in which the autoantibodies damage the tissues around the eyes. For instance, the fat, muscles and other soft tissues surrounding the eyes become inflamed and swollen, producing bulging, staring eyes.[4] Eye changes tend to be most severe in older men, although doctors are not sure why.[4] However, symptoms are usually mild, sometimes eye problems arise before doctors diagnose Graves' disease and, occasionally, orbitopathy is the only symptom of hyperthyroidism.[4]

Patients with Hashimoto's thyroiditis may develop more subtle eye changes than those with Graves's disease. However, retraction of the upper eyelid and mild inflammation are relatively common in people with Hashimoto's thyroiditis. For instance, in one study approximately one third of people with Hashimoto's thyroiditis developed eye changes. Of these, about a quarter had chronic retraction of the upper eyelid.[46]

Furthermore, the Royal National Institute of Blind People, which is an invaluable source of information and support, notes that treating an underlying thyroid condition can exacerbate orbitopathy. For example, radioiodine can exacerbate active eye disease,[4] especially among smokers.[24]

Difficult to diagnose

Bulging, staring eyes are a hallmark of Graves' disease. Nevertheless, thyroid eye disease can prove difficult to diagnose, especially when symptoms are relatively mild or affect only one eye. For example, doctors may mistakenly treat some people for conjunctivitis (inflammation of the outermost layer of the eye and the inner surface of the eyelids, triggered by, for example, chemical irritants, allergy or hay fever) for months or even years before eventually diagnosing thyroid orbitopathy.[4]

Doctors use several clues to help distinguish thyroid eye disease from other conditions, although you might need a scan to clinch the diagnosis (page 117). Remember that having thyroid disease does not protect you from developing other eye diseases simply by coincidence:

- Thyroid eye disease often causes symptoms all year round. Autumn and winter are generally the wrong seasons for hay fever. Nevertheless, some household allergic triggers, such as house dust mites and animal dander, may trigger conjunctivitis all year round.
- Unlike thyroid orbitopathy, allergies usually cause itchy eyes.
- Unlike thyroid orbitopathy, eye infections can cause sticky eyes. It is worth checking sticky eyes with your GP or pharmacist.
- Many people with thyroid eye disease experience aches or pain in or behind their eyes, especially when moving their eyes, and some report double vision. People with conjunctivitis, allergies or hay fever tend not to develop aches and pains around the eyes, or double vision. If you experience any of these symptoms, see a doctor or optician as soon as possible.

Dry eyes

The autoimmune attack around the eye can cause a wide range of symptoms, of which dry eyes are the most common. Autoantibodies (page 48) can attack the lacrimal gland, which then produces fewer tears, leaving your eyes feeling dry and gritty. Retraction of the eyelids and exophthalmos (which are discussed later in this chapter) often exacerbate dry eye. But ironically, dry eyes can make your eyes water a lot more than usual as the eyes try to compensate. People with dry eyes often find bright lights uncomfortable – a symptom known as photophobia. Lubricating eye drops (artificial tears) can make the eyes feel more comfortable and prevent damage.

Puffy eyes

Swollen tissue can hinder the drainage of fluid from the eye, which makes the upper eyelids even more puffy and helps to cause bags under the eyes.[4] Levothyroxine often improves the puffiness and some people find that sleeping with their head propped up with pillows helps. A diuretic (which increases the amount of fluid you lose in urine) may also reduce puffiness.[4]

Retraction of the eyelids

Contraction of the muscles in the eyelids pulls the lids back. Hyperthyroidism tends to cause the muscles in the upper eyelid to contract excessively, which exposes more of the white conjunctiva, making it look as though you are staring. In addition, the upper eyelids tend to lag behind the eyeballs' movement when you look down.[4]

Controlling hyperthyroidism reduces the eyelid retraction and the staring appearance in about two-thirds of people with Graves' orbitopathy. Some people also find that a beta-blocker (which relaxes the muscles in the eyelid) reduces retraction.[4]

Driving and double vision

Swollen muscles around the eyeball can mean your eyes move unequally, causing blurred or double vision. Driving with uncontrolled double vision is illegal. So if you develop double vision you must inform the Driver and Vehicle Licensing Authority (DVLA), which will probably contact your ophthalmologist. Prisms attached to spectacles, and steroids, which dampen the inflammation that causes the swollen muscle, can alleviate double vision. If glasses or an operation (see 'Long-term prospects' later in this chapter) control your double vision, the DVLA will probably declare you fit to drive. If in doubt, speak to your specialist, GP or the DVLA.

Exophthalmos

In some people, the swollen, inflamed muscles and fat can push the eyes forward so far that they bulge out of the sockets – a condition called exophthalmos.

Treating thyroid hyperactivity may improve exophthalmos in about 20 per cent of people with Graves' eye disease. However, any improvement is slow and the protrusion worsens in about 20 per cent of those treated. In the remainder, the exophthalmos remains the same.[4] So your doctor might suggest surgery to improve the appearance.

Meanwhile, you could wear sunglasses or tinted lenses. Dark eye shadow can help make the eyes recede and a bright lipstick or a striking top can draw attention away from your eyes.[7]

Visual loss

In severe orbitopathy, the increasing pressure exerted by the swollen tissue can squeeze the optic nerve. Over time, the pressure on the nerve can cause sight problems, such as dim vision, washed-out colours and a narrow visual field. To prevent permanent damage to your sight, seek medical help as soon as you notice a change in your vision or the way your eyes look, and have regular eye tests.

Younger people with exophthalmos are at especially high risk of developing sight problems. Their firmer tissues do not allow their eyes to bulge forward as easily as in middle-aged and elderly people. As a result, the pressure inside the sockets increases. Your doctor may suggest steroids or immunosuppressants (a group of drugs that dampen inflammation), radiotherapy or an operation called decompression surgery to reduce the pressure on the optic nerve and, hopefully, avoid permanent damage.

When to seek urgent help

See your doctor without delay and ask for referral if you experience any of the following:

- Symptoms that worsen over several days or weeks.
- Blurred vision that does not improve by blinking or covering each eye in turn.
- Colours that do not seem as bright as they used to.
- Colours that seem brighter when you close one eye.
- Double vision when you look forward or down.
- You have to keep your head tilted sideways or backwards to avoid double vision.

Long-term prospects

Mild eye changes often improve with treatment.[4] However, sometimes the changes are permanent and may need surgery.

Usually, the inflammation that causes thyroid orbitopathy burns out in about 2 years, the Royal National Institute of Blind People comments, and the eye problems gradually improve. For example, doctors from Newcastle-upon-Tyne followed 59 people with thyroid eye disease for, on average, a year. Of these, 22 per cent improved substantially and 42 per cent showed a minor improvement. Thyroid eye disease did not change in 22 per cent. Only about 14 per cent deteriorated to the point that they needed immunosuppressants.[47]

Nevertheless, retracted eyelids, exophthalmos or double vision can persist despite the burnt-out inflammation. Some ophthalmologists believe that low-dose radiotherapy early in the active phase of thyroid orbitopathy improves long-term prospects, and it's worth discussing this option. You may also need surgery to, for example, improve double vision and correct the lid position. Often a surgeon performs a series of operations over about 18 months to 2 years, once your thyroid disease is stable.

If you show marked exophthalmos or the pressure on the optic nerve threatens your vision, surgeons may remove a small amount of bone, fat or both so that the eye sits further back in its socket. However, this 'decompression' surgery may cause or exacerbate double vision and there is a small risk of serious sight problems.

Surgery can also correct permanent double vision caused by decompression surgery or thyroid disease. The surgeon lengthens the muscles to align the eyes, although this procedure can alter the position of the eyelids. As a result, you may need surgery to correct the position of the upper and lower eyelids so that you can close your eyes properly. A similar operation can correct eyelid retraction caused by the thyroid disease.

In other words, you might need operations not just to resolve the symptoms of thyroid eye disease but to correct the adverse effects of other operations. Nevertheless, operations on your eyes can be life-transforming, dramatically improve your appearance and even save your sight. So as I have mentioned several times, it's important to discuss the risks and benefits with your surgeon fully before embarking on what can be a long series of operations. It is also worth asking about the surgeon's success and complication rates, but as I have also mentioned before, bear in mind that the best surgeons often treat the most difficult cases.

Quit smoking for the sake of your eyes

Whether or not you have thyroid disease, quitting smoking is one of the best ways to protect your health generally and your sight in particular. Yet despite countless educational initiatives, numerous public health interventions and increasingly graphic warnings, about 1 in 5 adults in England still smoke. Indeed, smoking remains the single greatest cause of preventable illness and early death: according to the Department of Health, around half of those who do not quit smoking die prematurely.

Cancer is, perhaps, the best known of the numerous diseases caused by smoking. The German physician Samuel Thomas von Sömmering noted a link between pipe smoking and lip cancer in 1795.[48] We now know that smoking caused 86 per cent of lung cancers in the UK during 2010 as well as, among other malignancies:

- 65 per cent of cancers in the mouth, throat and oesophagus;
- 29 per cent of pancreatic cancers;
- 22 per cent of stomach cancers.[49]

Overall, smokers are roughly twice as likely to die from cancer as non-smokers.

The dangers to your family of smoking

If the harm smoking does to your health is not enough to make you quit, think of the harm you are doing to your loved ones. According to the National Cancer Institute in the USA, tobacco smoke contains more than 7,000 chemicals. More than 250 of these are harmful, including at least 69 carcinogens (cancer-causing chemicals). Second-hand smoke contains more than 4,000 chemicals, about 50 of which are carcinogens. This chemical cocktail increases the risk that people who inhale second-hand smoke will develop serious diseases, including cancer, heart disease, asthma, sudden infant death syndrome and, according to some studies, thyroid disease. For example, the risks that a woman who has never smoked will develop lung cancer and heart disease are 24 and 30 per cent greater respectively, if she lives with a smoker.

Smoking also damages your cardiovascular system, which is bad news for anyone. For example, smoking roughly trebles your chances of having a stroke and causes around half of all cases of heart disease, independently of thyroid disease. The other cardio-vascular conditions linked to thyroid problems mean that smoking is especially dangerous for your heart and circulatory system if you have thyroid disease.

Smoking and eye disease

Smoking causes or exacerbates several eye diseases:

- According to Action on Smoking and Health (ASH), people who smoke at least 20 cigarettes a day are twice as likely to develop cataracts as lifelong non-smokers. Cataracts arise from clouding in the lens in the eye, which can lead to blurred vision and, if untreated, sight loss.
- Age-related macular degeneration (AMD) refers to damage in the macula, a tiny area of the light-sensitive retina, which is responsible for the clear, central vision you use to read, drive and watch television. Smoking is the most important preventable cause of AMD, which, ASH notes, is the leading cause of blindness in people over 65 years of age in the Western world.
- People with type 1 diabetes are at increased risk of developing thyroid disease and are vulnerable to diabetic retinopathy, which occurs when high levels of sugar damage the vessels that supply blood to the back of the eye. The cells do not receive sufficient oxygen and nutrients and so die. ASH notes that smoking can hasten or worsen diabetic retinopathy by further damaging blood vessels.

Smoking and thyroid disease

Smoking seems to increase the risk of several thyroid diseases. In one study, researchers asked 617 patients with hyperthyroidism and 408 with autoimmune hypothyroidism in Denmark about their smoking habits. They then compared each patient to a randomly selected healthy person of the same age and sex.[50]

Women who smoked were 150 per cent more likely to develop Graves' disease, 70 per cent more likely to develop toxic nodular goitre and 50 per cent more likely to develop autoimmune hypothyroidism compared with those who never smoked. Indeed, smoking could directly or indirectly cause 45 per cent of Graves' disease cases, 28 per cent of toxic nodular goitres and 23 per cent of cases of autoimmune hypothyroidism. However, smoking did not seem to increase the risk of thyroid disease in men.[50]

Smoking also dramatically increases the risk of developing thyroid eye disease. For example, fewer than 1 in 10 non- or ex-smokers with Graves' disease who did not experience eye problems before the doctor diagnosed the thyroid disease go on to develop orbitopathy. Heavy smokers with Graves' disease, the British Thyroid Foundation warns, are eight times more likely to develop thyroid eye disease than non-smokers. Doctors do not yet fully understand the link between smoking and thyroid eye disease. However, smoking may impair the immune system, which might contribute.

To make matters worse, people with thyroid eye disease who smoke respond less well to treatments. For example, carbimazole or propylthiouracil are more likely to resolve hyperthyroidism in non-smokers or ex-smokers than smokers. However, this disadvantage seems to disappear rapidly after quitting.

Making quitting easier

Quitting reduces the risk of most smoking-related diseases. According to the Department of Health, an average lifelong smoker dies about 10 years sooner than they would otherwise. A person who stops smoking at 30 or 40 years of age gains, on average, 10 and 9 years of life, respectively. Even a 60-year-old gains 3 years by quitting.

Unfortunately, on some measures, nicotine is more addictive than heroin or cocaine. In the 2007 report *Harm Reduction in Nicotine Addiction*, the Royal College of Physicians noted that compared with cocaine, heroin and other drugs of abuse, 'initial use of nicotine is more likely to lead to addictive use'.

Nicotine's potent addictive qualities help to explain why, while 67 per cent of smokers would like to stop, only about 4 per cent manage to quit for at least a year without support. NHS stop-smoking services increase the proportion who quit for at least a year to 15 per cent. Unfortunately, more than half start smoking again within a year.

In the early days after quitting, intense withdrawal symptoms can leave you irritable, restless and anxious, experiencing insomnia and intensely craving a cigarette. These symptoms generally abate over 2 weeks or so. If you cannot tough it out, nicotine replacement therapy (NRT) tops up nicotine levels in the blood without exposing you to the other harmful chemicals in tobacco. This alleviates the withdrawal symptoms and increases your chances of quitting by between 50 and 100 per cent.

Drugs to help you quit smoking

There are now several types of NRT, so you should be able to find one that meets your needs:

- Patches reduce withdrawal symptoms over a relatively long time, but have a slow onset of action.
- Nicotine chewing gum, lozenges, inhalers and nasal sprays act more quickly than patches.
- The National Institute for Health and Care Excellence (NICE) advocates replacing each cigarette with a licensed NRT, such as a lozenge or piece of gum. NRT releases nicotine more slowly than a cigarette. Ideally, smokers should use NRT before the usual time they would have smoked.

Doctors can prescribe other treatments, such as bupropion and varenicline, to help you quit. You could also try e-cigarettes, which are now regulated in the same way as other forms of NRT. Talk to your pharmacist or GP to find the right treatment or combination for you.

NICE comments that NRT is safe for at least 5 years and adds that 'there is reason to believe that lifetime use of licensed nicotine-containing products will be considerably less harmful than smoking'. However, some studies have raised concerns that smoking cessation therapies might increase the risk of events linked to cardiovascular disease, such as arrhythmias, heart attacks and so on. Nevertheless, a recent paper considered 67 studies and found that neither bupropion nor varenicline increased the risk of cardiovascular disease. NRT roughly doubled the risk of cardiovascular events, but these were mainly less serious events such as tachycardia (a fast heartbeat), which, the authors comment, is 'well-known and largely benign'. There's no evidence that smoking cessation therapies increase the risk of serious cardiovascular events. In other words, NRT is a lot better for your heart than smoking – but quitting is even better.

Tips to help you quit

While smoking cessation treatments offer a helping hand, you still need to be motivated to quit. A few simple hints may make life easier:

- Set a quit date when you will stop completely. Smokers are more likely to quit if they set a specific date rather than saying, for example, that they will give up in the next 2 months.

- Quit abruptly. People who cut back the number of cigarettes they smoke usually inhale more deeply to get the same amount of nicotine. Nevertheless, cutting back seems to increase the likelihood that you will eventually quit by, in some studies, 70 per cent compared with those who never cut back. So while reduction takes you a step towards kicking the habit, do not stop there.

- Plan ahead. For a couple of weeks before you quit, keep a diary of problems and situations that tempt you to light up, such as stress, coffee, meals, pubs or work breaks. Understanding when and why you light up helps you find alternatives or how to avoid the cue.

- Try to find something to take your mind off smoking. If you find yourself smoking when you get home in the evening, try a new hobby or exercise. If you find car journeys boring without a cigarette, try an audio book. Most people find that the craving for a cigarette usually only lasts a couple of minutes.

- Smoking is expensive. Keep a note of how much you save and spend at least some of it on something for yourself.

- Tackle stress. Try relaxation therapies (page 121), exercise (page 117) or take up a hobby that you enjoy.

- Ask if your area offers NHS antismoking clinics, which offer advice, support and, when appropriate, NRT. You can also obtain a free quit-smoking support pack from the NHS Smoking Helpline (0800 022 4332).

- Hypnosis can increase your chances of quitting smoking almost fivefold.[51] Ask your doctor for a recommendation or contact the British Association of Medical Hypnosis.

- Deal with hunger pangs without reaching for the sweet packet, which may mean you put on weight. On average, people who quit smoking without treatment gained 1.12 kg (2.47 lbs) during the month after quitting and 4.67 kg (10.3 lbs) after a year.[52] However, 16 per cent of people *lost* weight after quitting and 37 per cent gained less than 5 kg (11 lbs). Only 13 per cent gained more than 10 kg (22 lbs).[52] Try our weight-loss tips on page 108.

Dealing with setbacks

As we have seen, nicotine is incredibly addictive and, not surprisingly, most people do not quit the first time they try. Indeed, Andrew Russell points out that most smokers make three or four attempts to quit before they succeed. Try to regard any relapse as a temporary setback, set another quit date and try again. It is also worth trying to identify why you relapsed. Were you stressed out? If so, why? Was smoking linked to a particular time, place or event? Once you know why you slipped you can develop strategies to stop the problem in the future. So as the old health promotion advertisement suggests, 'Don't give up on giving up'.

Try selenium to protect your sight

Selenium supplements may improve mild thyroid eye disease. A European study compared a selenium supplement with an inactive placebo in 104 people with mild Graves' orbitopathy. Neither patients nor doctors knew whether the treatment was the supplement or the placebo.

After 6 months, Graves' orbitopathy improved in 61 per cent of those taking selenium compared with 36 per cent for placebo. Eye disease worsened in 7 per cent of those taking selenium and 26 per cent of the placebo group. Selenium also seemed to improve vision, reduce the distance between the eyelids, ameliorate the soft tissue changes and enhance quality of life.[53] It might be worth discussing taking selenium supplements with your doctor. However, as ever, always check with your doctor before taking supplements if you are on any other medication.

Eye changes are undoubtedly one of the more distressing and readily apparent symptoms of thyroid disease. Unfortunately, eye changes are also one of the more difficult changes to treat: improving your appearance and ameliorating the symptoms might involve a long series of operations. Nevertheless, try not to lose heart; there's a lot you and your medical teams can do to improve thyroid eye disease.

7

Thyroid cancer

Every 3–4 hours, someone in the UK receives the devastating news that they have thyroid cancer. Overall, about 1 in 100 people develops thyroid cancer.[32] During 2010, doctors diagnosed about 1,900 women and 700 men in the UK with thyroid cancer, according to Cancer Research UK. Almost half were under 50 years of age. Thyroid cancer is also the third most common solid cancer in children. (Solid cancers do not include malignancies of blood, bone marrow and lymph nodes, such as leukaemia, lymphoma and myeloma.) Overall, between 5 and 10 per cent of thyroid cancers occur in children.[18]

Nodules and cancer

In general, goitres do not seem to increase the risk of thyroid cancer: most malignancies seem to develop in previously normal glands.[4] Nevertheless, about 1 in 20 nodules prove to be cancerous.[31] For instance, in a recent study, about 2 per cent of people with at least one nodule with a diameter of 5 mm or more on an ultrasound scan had thyroid cancer.[32] Thyroid nodules are especially likely to be malignant in:

- Men
- People who have undergone radiotherapy to their head or neck
- Children
- Adults who are under 30 or over 60 years of age.[31]

Worryingly, thyroid cancer seems to be becoming more common. For example, doctors from the USA reported that between 1997 and 2005, the number of tumours with a diameter less than 1 cm increased by about 10 per cent a year in men and by 9 per cent in women. The number of cancers over 4 cm in diameter increased by almost 4 per cent each year in men and by 6 per cent in women over the same period. The increase in larger cancers (which would be noticed with older methods) suggests that better detection is not solely responsible for the greater number of thyroid cancers.[54]

But there is some good news: the chances of survival are improving. During the 1970s, half of people with thyroid cancer survived for at least 5 years, compared with about three-quarters today. Indeed, more than 95 per cent of people aged less than 40 years with thyroid cancer now survive for at least 5 years, although the course is less predictable in older people.[16] During 2010, around 130 men and 210 women died from thyroid cancer in the UK.

Types of thyroid cancer

Thyroid cancer is not a single disease. Doctors recognize several subtypes. In addition, each subtype develops, if untreated, through various stages, from changes that are barely discernible under the microscope to a lump several centimetres across. You can learn more about the staging of thyroid cancer on the Cancer Research UK website (see 'Useful addresses').

The most common thyroid malignancies – papillary and medullary cancers – are 'differentiated'. In other words, the cancer resembles and acts similarly to normal thyroid cells, although they are different enough to distinguish under the microscope and on certain diagnostic tests. Undifferentiated cells, which can include lymphoma (a cancer arising from a type of white blood cell) or metastases (cancer that has spread to or from another part of the body), look and behave markedly differently from normal thyroid cells.[4]

Papillary tumours

Papillary tumours account for about 60–85 per cent of cancers in the thyroid gland. Doctors usually discover papillary thyroid carcinoma when investigating nodules. According to Cancer Research UK, papillary tumours typically emerge in younger people and women. Often the cancer begins in one of the gland's lobes and is usually painless. Sometimes enlarged lymph nodes may be the first sign of papillary thyroid cancer.

The malignancy tends to grow slowly, and provided doctors diagnose papillary cancer early, while the tumour is small and confined to the gland, 99 per cent of patients survive at least 5 years after diagnosis. However, late recurrences can occur and you should remain alert for any sign of the cancer and attend your appointments.

Follicular tumours

Doctors usually diagnose follicular thyroid cancer in middle-aged people. The prognosis for this malignancy, which accounts for about 15 per cent of thyroid cancers, is also relatively good: with early diagnosis, about 98 per cent of patients survive at least 5 years.

Medullary tumours

Medullary malignancies arise in C cells (page 16) and account for between 5 and 8 per cent of thyroid cancers.[54] Cancer Research UK notes that approximately a quarter of these malignancies arise from a faulty gene inherited from a biological parent (page 24). Benign (non-cancerous) tumours in the parathyroid or adrenal gland also seem to be linked to an increased risk of medullary thyroid cancer.[4]

Anaplastic tumours

Anaplastic malignancies, which account for less than 2 per cent of thyroid cancers, arise from follicles (page 4). Anaplastic cancers usually grow more rapidly than other malignancies in the thyroid gland. According to Cancer Research UK, three-quarters of people with anaplastic thyroid cancer are over 60 years of age and, as we have seen time and time again with thyroid disease, the malignancy is more common in women than men.

The anaplastic cells are even more abnormal than other malignancies affecting the thyroid. For example, anaplastic cells do not take up iodine or make thyroglobulin. Although rare, anaplastic thyroid cancer is one of the most aggressive cancers of any site:[54] only between 10 and 20 per cent of people are still alive 5 years after diagnosis.[55]

Other thyroid cancers

A variety of other malignancies can arise in the thyroid:

- Poorly differentiated thyroid cancer (a mix of different subtypes) accounts for 1–6 per cent of malignancies in the gland.[54]
- Very rarely, non-Hodgkin's lymphoma develops in the thyroid. About half of these patients have previously developed Hashimoto's thyrotoxicosis.[4]
- Occasionally, a malignant cell from a cancer elsewhere in the body (typically in a lung, breast or kidney) can lead to a thyroid tumour.[4] In these cases, the thyroid gland is a site of metastases.

Risk factors for thyroid cancer

Several factors increase the risk of thyroid cancer, including radiation being female or overweight, and even sleep disturbances.[56,57] For example, in a recent study, obesity increased the risk of thyroid cancer by 63 per cent in women and by 16 per cent in men, after allowing for age, smoking and TSH levels. However, the authors could not rule out that the increased risk in men was due to chance. Furthermore, the study did not include people with a family history of thyroid cancer.[58]

Some families seem to be particularly prone to developing thyroid cancer, indicating that genes (page 24) carry some of the risk.[55] For example, an abnormal gene known as the *RET* proto-oncogene increases the risk of medullary thyroid cancer. If a close relative develops medullary thyroid cancer or has the *RET* proto-oncogene, your GP can refer you for genetic tests. You may opt for regular testing or an operation to remove the cancer-prone gland.

RET and MEN2

We discussed genes in Chapter 3. A proto-oncogene is a normal gene that can trigger cancer when damage causes it to change (mutate) or become overactive. One proto-oncogene, known as *RET*, increases the chance of developing a condition called multiple endocrine neoplasia type 2 (MEN2). People with MEN2 are more likely to develop malignancies in their glands, including thyroid cancer. Medullary thyroid cancer usually develops at a young age in people carrying a version of the gene that causes a subtype of the condition called MEN2B. If this gene runs in your family, doctors now test children and may suggest a thyroidectomy to prevent the cancer.

Radiation and thyroid cancer

Radiation is probably the best-studied risk factor for thyroid cancer:

- Researchers linked a peak in the number of thyroid cancers in women in England and Wales born between 1952 and 1955 with fallout from worldwide testing of nuclear weapons. The number of thyroid cancers was especially high in parts of Wales that received the greatest amount of nuclear fallout.[56]
- In 1986, the Chernobyl nuclear accident released large amounts of radioactive caesium and iodine. The radioactive iodine con-

taminated milk and, about 5 years later, the number of cases of thyroid cancer began rising dramatically in people living near the plant, especially among children. By 1995, 40 children per million under the age of 10 years in the worst-affected areas (Belarus, Ukraine and four Russian Federation regions) developed thyroid cancer each year. This compared with between 1 and 5 per million annually in the USA.[59]

- People working in the nuclear industry, radiologists and the military are especially likely to be exposed to radiation and, therefore, develop thyroid cancer. Aircraft cabin crew also seem to be at increased risk: the atmosphere, which blocks radiation from space, is thinner at 30,000 feet than at sea level.[55]

However, thyroid cancer may not emerge until 40 years after exposure to radiation.[18] You probably need one or more additional risk factors, such as another mutation or obesity, to trigger the cancer's development.

Sleep problems and thyroid cancer

Intriguingly, sleep disturbances may contribute to thyroid cancer. Researchers in America looked at 142,933 women aged between 50 and 79 years. Over the next 11 years, about 1 in 500 developed thyroid cancer. After the researchers had allowed for other risk factors, women who suffered from insomnia were 71 per cent more likely to develop thyroid cancer than those who slept well, but only if they were not obese. Sleep disturbances did not seem to increase the risk of thyroid cancer in obese women.[57] Doctors do not know why obese people are not at increased risk from the sleep disturbance. Possibly, the increased risk of developing cancer that is associated with obesity alone 'overwhelms' the increase linked to thyroid disease.

Indeed, researchers do not understand why insomnia may increase the risk of thyroid disease. There are several possibilities:

- Sleep disturbances might undermine the immune system's ability to attack malignancies.
- Sleep disturbances might increase TSH levels, which could increase the risk by overstimulating growth of the thyroid gland.
- Daytime tiredness might reduce the amount of exercise people take. Exercise (page 117) seems to protect against several cancers.
- Insomnia may change levels of hormones that regulate appetite.

So sleep disturbances may promote weight gain. Indeed, obesity and lack of exercise increase the risk of several cancers.[57]

Although the link is not definite, and while the reason remains uncertain, the study underscores the value of a good night's sleep – see our tips on page 113.

Treating thyroid cancer

Surgery to remove all, or almost all, of the gland – total or near-total thyroidectomy – is the mainstay of thyroid cancer treatment and effectively cures many malignancies. In some cases, the surgeon may also remove lymph nodes near to the gland. The cancer can use the lymph (page 2) to spread to other parts of the body (metastases). However, if you have developed a single, small and relatively low-risk cancer, the surgeon may remove only the tumour and a margin of healthy tissue surrounding the gland. You will be monitored to make sure no cancer remains.

Assuming that the surgeon is experienced at thyroidectomy, only about 1 or 2 per cent of people experience complications. These can include hypoparathyroidism (underproduction of parathyroid hormone; page 7) and laryngeal nerve palsy – damage to an important nerve supplying the larynx.[54] If the surgeon damages this nerve, the person's voice may change (page 60) and she or he may experience breathing problems.

You will also usually receive radioiodine, with the aim of destroying any remaining cancerous tissue, even if the tumours are microscopic or have spread to the lymph nodes or other parts of the body, such as the lungs, bone, liver and brain. Metastases may retain some characteristics of the original cancer, including the ability to take up radioiodine.[54] Your doctor will probably treat you with TSH before administering radioiodine to make sure the cells take up as much radioactive iodine as possible.[54]

Your doctor will suggest regular testing to ensure that replacement treatment with levothyroxine (page 42) is effective and to watch for signs that the cancer might have recurred:

• Levothyroxine suppresses the production of TSH, which can stimulate thyroid cells, including those that are malignant, to grow. Doctors may look for thyroglobulin (page 4) in your blood as a sign of recurrence.[54]

- Medullary thyroid cancers release several proteins, including calcitonin (page 6). Increased calcitonin levels in the blood after surgery might indicate that the cancer has recurred or spread to another part of your body.[54]

Unfortunately, the outlook for people who develop metastatic thyroid cancer is worse than if doctors treat the malignancy early. Nevertheless, it is still better than many other metastatic malignancies:

- According to Cancer Research UK, around half of people with metastatic (stage 4) follicular cancer live for at least 5 years.
- Between 25 and 40 per cent of people with metastatic medullary cancer live for at least 5 years.
- By way of contrast, only 4 per cent of adults with pancreatic cancer (the pancreas is the gland that makes insulin) survive for at least 5 years.

Your cancer team will tailor treatment to alleviate the symptoms produced by metastases.

Drugs for thyroid cancer

Traditionally, there were few drugs for metastatic thyroid cancer.[54] However, several clinical studies are underway. One study included 417 people with locally recurrent (re-emerged in and around the gland) or metastatic progressive differentiated thyroid cancer that did not respond to radioiodine. Sorafenib – a drug used to treat certain kidney and liver cancers – increased the time patients lived without the cancer getting worse (progression-free survival) by 41 per cent. Half of the patients receiving sorafenib lived without their cancer progressing for at least 10.8 months, compared with at least 5.8 months for people who received an inactive placebo.

Another drug, called vemurafenib, currently used to treat melanoma (a type of cancer that usually emerges in the skin), is showing promise in papillary thyroid cancer. About half of people with papillary thyroid cancer have a change in a gene called *BRAFV600E*. Vemurafenib targets the protein produced by this gene and so works only in people with this mutation.

However, these treatments are, at the time of writing, experimental. And there are many clinical trials that assess other new treatments. If you would like to take part, speak to your cancer team or contact Cancer Research UK or Macmillan Cancer Support for further information.

8

Thyroid problems and pregnancy

Pregnancy, even when everything goes smoothly, places considerable demands on your body. In response, your thyroid gland increases its activity to help your body keep up. As a result, your thyroid gland usually enlarges by up to almost a third between the 18th and 36th weeks of pregnancy. Ancient Egyptian newlyweds used to tie a reed or thread around the bride's neck. When it snapped, it was a sign she was pregnant.[7]

Your increasingly active thyroid is one of several reasons why you need to make sure your diet contains sufficient nutrients, including iodine, to keep you and your developing baby healthy. You need up to 50 per cent more iodine during pregnancy and when breastfeeding than at other times of your life.[11] This makes sure that the developing baby gets sufficient iodine to ensure normal development. Severe lack of iodine often left children severely mentally and physically disabled, a condition called cretinism. Fortunately, this is now extremely rare in the UK. However, even mild iodine deficiency during pregnancy can leave your baby with a lower IQ or worse school performance than his or her classmates.[10,11] Recent research suggests that two-thirds of women in the UK do not get enough iodine during pregnancy.[10]

Indeed, thyroid problems are common among women of child-bearing age. Even subclinical hypothyroidism seems to increase the risk of complications before, during and after birth. For example, subclinical hypothyroidism in early pregnancy increases the risk of pre-eclampsia (dangerously increased blood pressure and high levels of protein in your urine) by 70 per cent.[60] Pre-eclampsia can cause serious problems for mother and baby, including life-threatening fits. Once they have given birth, some women show hyperthyroidism followed, as the gland becomes depleted of thyroid hormone, by hypothyroidism. Doctors call this condition postpartum thyroiditis.

Sometimes such problems emerge in women without a history of thyroid disease. Between 8 and 14 per cent of women of fertile age produce antibodies against thyroid peroxidase (page 16) or thyroglobulin (page 4), but show normal thyroid function.[61] Doctors believe that the antibodies damage the gland, leaving the thyroid unable to respond adequately to the increasing demands during pregnancy, even if the mother-to-be does not normally experience symptoms.[60]

Nevertheless, if you have a history of thyroid disease, speak to your doctor before becoming pregnant. (So it's a good idea to use reliable contraception until the doctor lets you know if it is safe to try for a baby.) If you are at high risk – such as having a sibling with thyroid disease – you might want to discuss having further tests with your doctor when you decide to have a baby.

Thyroid disease and infertility

Unfortunately, thyroid disease can cause problems even before you know you are pregnant. About 8–12 per cent of couples trying to conceive for the first time are infertile. The woman and the man are about equally likely to be infertile.

Carl von Basedow noted in 1840 that Graves' disease could influence menstruation. Today, we know that both hypo- and hyperthyroidism can affect your periods. While hypothyroidism can lead to light, scanty periods, an overactive thyroid can cause very heavy periods. Severe hypothyroidism can also stop you from releasing an egg each month ('anovulation').[7] Obviously, if you do not release an egg you cannot conceive.

Furthermore, women with thyroid antibodies are about 50 per cent more likely to experience difficulties conceiving than women without autoimmune reactions against the gland.[60] Antithyroid drugs usually rapidly restore normal menstruation and fertility.[4] So if you have trouble conceiving after a few months, you might want to ask your doctor for a thyroid function test.

Mild iodine deficiency

Your baby needs iodine from the start of pregnancy. As a result, the British Dietetic Association suggests ensuring that you get at least 150 µg of iodine each day for several months before you conceive. This bolsters your stores. As your breasts concentrate iodine, you also need more iodine from your diet when breastfeeding.[11]

Iodine supplements

If you are pregnant or breastfeeding, the British Dietetic Association suggests that you take a multivitamin and mineral supplement containing 140 or 150 μg iodine. Your diet should make up the difference (you need about 250 μg). Choose a supplement specifically designed for pregnant or breastfeeding women. You can also boost your intake of iodine-rich foods (page 95).

It is hard to overstate how important it is to get sufficient iodine during pregnancy and while breastfeeding. In adults, treatment can reverse many of the problems caused by hypothyroidism. But hypothyroidism and insufficient iodine from the diet during pregnancy can cause permanent abnormalities in a baby. Indeed, iodine deficiency remains the main cause of preventable intellectual disability worldwide.[9]

Iodine and mental development

Although cretinism is now rare in the UK, even mild iodine deficiency can undermine mental development. Australian researchers, for example, compared the educational attainment of children whose mothers experienced mild iodine deficiency during pregnancy with those of mothers who received recommended levels. At 9 years of age, children born to mothers with mild iodine deficiency showed worse spelling (10 per cent reduction in scores), grammar (7.6 per cent) and English literacy (5.7 per cent). The children received sufficient iodine in their diet. However, this did not make up for the low levels they received while in the womb.[11]

Similar results emerged in a UK study. About 67 per cent of women were iodine deficient during pregnancy. The researchers divided IQ and reading ability into four groups, called quartiles:

- Children born to women who were iodine deficient during pregnancy were 58 per cent more likely to have scores in the lowest quartile for verbal IQ at 8 years of age than those born to women who were not iodine deficient: 29 and 20 per cent of children, respectively, were in the lowest quartile.
- At 9 years of age, children born to women who were iodine deficient during pregnancy were 69 per cent more likely to have

scores in the lowest quartile for reading accuracy than those born to women who were not iodine deficient (29 and 19 per cent, respectively).

- At 9 years of age, children born to women who were iodine deficient during pregnancy were 54 per cent more likely to have scores in the lowest quartile for reading comprehension than those born to women who were not iodine deficient (30 and 21 per cent, respectively).[10]

Severe hypothyroidism during pregnancy may also increase the risk of autism. Researchers found severe hypothyroidism in approximately 3 per cent of 5,100 women tested after, on average, 13 weeks' pregnancy. Eighty children assessed at 6 years of age had probable autism (doctors cannot make a definitive diagnosis until later life). Babies born to women with severe hypothyroidism during pregnancy were almost four times as likely to be diagnosed with probable autism than those born to women with normal thyroid function.[62]

Thyroid disease during pregnancy

As Table 8.1 shows, thyroid problems are common among women of childbearing age. In 85 per cent of cases, hyperthyroidism during pregnancy arises from Graves' disease (page 47). However, both hyper- and hypothyroidism can cause complications before, during and after giving birth. Some of these complications are listed in Table 8.2. For example, women with thyroid antibodies are at roughly twice the risk of recurrent miscarriage (2.3 times) and premature birth (1.9 times), and almost four times (3.7 times) more likely to miscarry at least once.[60] If you are worried, speak to your doctor or midwife.

Table 8.1 Thyroid problems in pregnancy

Disease	Percentage of pregnant women
Subclinical hypothyroidism	3–5
Thyroid disease	2–3
Hypothyroidism	0.3–0.5
Hyperthyroidism	0.1–0.4

Source: Based on Vissenberg et al.[61]

Table 8.2 Possible complications from thyroid disease during pregnancy

---

Hyperthyroidism

    Miscarriage

    Premature birth

    Pre-eclampsia

Hypothyroidism

    Miscarriage

    Anaemia during pregnancy

    Pre-eclampsia

    Heavy bleeding after giving birth

    Premature birth

    Low birth weight

Source: Based on Lazarus[41]

Treating thyroid disease during pregnancy

Effective treatment can markedly reduce the risk of many complications that can arise from thyroid disease during pregnancy. For example:

- In women with hypothyroidism, levothyroxine reduces the risk of miscarriage by 81 per cent and premature birth by 59 per cent.[61]
- In women with hyperthyroidism, propylthiouracil reduces the risk of premature birth and pre-eclampsia by 77 per cent and low birth weight by 62 per cent.[61]

As we have seen, being pregnant increases demands on your thyroid. As a result, your doctor may suggest altering your treatment during pregnancy. However, some women find that thyroid disease improves during pregnancy.

Just under half the genes in your baby come from the father (page 25) and is, therefore, 'foreign' tissue. Indeed, a fetus is so different that in other circumstances the body would mount an immune attack. However, the body recognizes that the baby is a special case and the activity of some elements of your immune system declines during pregnancy. As a result, autoimmune reactions tend to weaken in the later stages of pregnancy. In response, your doctor may reduce the dose or even stop antithyroid treatment during the third trimester. Unfortunately, most women with Graves' disease relapse 3–6 months after giving birth.[24]

Carbimazole and unborn babies

You need to discuss with your doctor the risks and benefits of any treatment – for your baby and yourself – that you take during pregnancy. Carbimazole, for example, crosses the placenta. In general, assuming the dose is within the standard range and thyroid function is monitored, carbimazole does not seem to increase the risk that the baby will be born with abnormalities in his or her thyroid. In general, the risk of congenital malformations (birth defects) is greater if the mother's hyperthyroidism is untreated than it is for those who receive carbimazole.

Nevertheless, in rare cases, congenital malformations can occur with carbimazole during pregnancy. These malformations can arise in the kidney, skull, cardiovascular system, eyes, gastrointestinal tract and umbilical cord.

Propylthiouracil, by contrast, does not seem to cause these abnormalities.[24] Therefore, doctors use carbimazole in pregnancy only when propylthiouracil is unsuitable, and they prescribe the lowest effective dose. They may also discontinue carbimazole 3–4 weeks before your baby's expected date of birth to reduce the risk of problems in your newborn baby.

Radioiodine and pregnancy

Radioiodine does not seem to increase the risks of malformation, provided you do not become pregnant within 6 months of treatment.[24] Doctors generally recommend avoiding pregnancy for 6–12 months after treatment with radioiodine for cancer to ensure that the thyroid function is stable or the malignancy is in remission.[4]

Monitoring thyroid function in pregnancy

Your doctor may suggest monitoring your thyroid function more regularly during pregnancy. For example, mothers-to-be with Graves' disease will probably need monitoring at least every 4 weeks.[24]

However, doctors cannot use the reference range (page 15) for thyroid function tests they used when you were not pregnant. During pregnancy, the level of thyroxine-binding globulin in the blood almost doubles. As we have seen, this protein carries T_3 and T_4 around the body. So levels of thyroid hormone rise to ensure that free levels can meet the body's demands.

Furthermore, you probably tested whether you were pregnant using a home test. Most pregnancy tests detect levels of human chorionic gonadotropin (hCG) – a hormone made by the fertilized egg and placenta – in your urine. However, hCG can stimulate the TSH receptor, causing transient gestational thyrotoxicosis, which generally resolves once you give birth.[41]

Because hCG stimulates the TSH receptor, blood levels of TSH decline during the first trimester. The decline is particularly marked in women who have twins or another multiple pregnancy, and blood levels of TSH are occasionally completely suppressed in a normal pregnancy. So doctors will evaluate your thyroid function using TSH and T_4 ranges that are specific for each trimester.[4,25]

Thyroiditis after giving birth

Overall, between 5 and 7 per cent of women worldwide develop postpartum thyroiditis.[22] However, women with thyroid antibodies are 11.5 times more likely to develop postpartum thyroiditis than those without the autoimmune reaction.[60] People with other autoimmune diseases are also at increased risk of postpartum thyroiditis. For example, at least 15 per cent of women with type 1 diabetes develop postpartum thyroiditis.[22] Doctors can mistake hypothyroidism's often subtle symptoms and signs for other illnesses – including postnatal depression – in women who have recently given birth.[25]

According to the British Thyroid Foundation, postpartum thyroiditis usually emerges in the first 6 months after giving birth. New mums with postpartum thyroiditis find that their thyroid is slightly swollen, although the enlarged gland is almost never painful. Initially, women develop symptoms of hyperthyroidism, which in some cases resolves. But some women go on to develop symptoms of hypothyroidism (page 34).

Doctors diagnose postpartum thyroiditis using a combination of physical examination and blood tests for thyroid hormones and antibodies. In some cases, doctors may suggest a radioisotope uptake scan (page 19) to help confirm the diagnosis. You will need to interrupt breastfeeding for a few days.

Mild postpartum thyroiditis can clear up quickly without treatment. In other cases, a doctor may prescribe a beta-blocker (page 10) to treat troublesome symptoms of hyperthyroidism or levothyroxine to alleviate hypothyroidism. The British Thyroid Foundation notes that neither beta-blockers nor levothyroxine interferes with breastfeeding. However, always check with a doctor or pharmacist before taking any drug – whether prescribed or bought without a prescription – if you are pregnant or breastfeeding.

Many women with postpartum thyroiditis can stop levothyroxine after 6–12 months, following discussions with their doctor. However, about half still have hypothyroidism a year after giving birth and will probably need further treatment.[22]

Postpartum thyroiditis may recur after subsequent pregnancies. So you need to let your midwife and doctor know when you know you are pregnant. They will arrange a thyroid test, usually 2–3 months after each birth. In addition, women who developed postpartum thyroiditis are more likely to develop permanent thyroid disease. As a result, the British Thyroid Foundation suggests having blood tests once a year to check thyroid function.

Smoking, breastfeeding and the thyroid

Smoking while you are breastfeeding is bad for you and your baby – for numerous reasons. You can pass some cancer-causing chemicals to your baby in your breast milk. Furthermore, tobacco smoke contains large amounts of a chemical called thiocyanate, which can halve the amount of iodine in breast milk.[2]

Thyroid disease in newborns

The antibodies that cause Graves' disease can cross the placenta and bind to and stimulate TSH receptors (page 9) in the developing baby's thyroid. Overall, between 1 and 5 per cent of babies born to women with Graves' disease have hyperthyroidism.

As a result, doctors monitor the babies of mothers-to-be with Graves' disease especially carefully. For example, a very fast heart rate, slow growth or a goitre seen on an ultrasound scan may suggest that the baby has hyperthyroidism. The baby can receive an antithyroid drug, which crosses the placenta, while the mother takes levothyroxine, which does not cross the placenta to any significant extent, to avoid hypothyroidism.[4]

Congenital hypothyroidism

About 1 in every 3,500 children born in the UK has congenital hypothyroidism. In about 80 per cent of cases, according to the British Society for Paediatric Endocrinology and Diabetes (BSPED), the thyroid gland does not develop properly. Doctors call this dysgenesis. The other babies with congenital hypothyroidism show abnormal production of thyroid hormone – so-called thyroid dyshormonogenesis (page 26).

A baby with congenital hypothyroidism often seems normal and healthy at birth. The physical and behavioural problems arising from the lack of thyroid hormone may not emerge for several weeks. However, irreversible damage to the brain and other organs may arise by the time physical and behavioural problems develop. So around the fifth day after birth, a midwife takes a small blood sample, by pricking the baby's heel, to detect a range of problems including sickle cell disease, cystic fibrosis and congenital hypothyroidism.

If the heel test detects a possibility of congenital hypothyroidism, doctors will test another blood sample more accurately. If this confirms congenital hypothyroidism, treatment with levothyroxine begins immediately. The doctor may also suggest a scan to help identify the cause.

Obviously, learning that your baby has congenital hypothyroidism is distressing and worrying. However, the BSPED comments that provided treatment with levothyroxine begins in the first few weeks after birth, the child's growth and development are 'almost always' normal.

Your doctor will tell you the best way to give your baby levothyroxine. That may be a liquid version or crushing a tablet and mixing the levothyroxine in milk. But whichever way you agree with your doctor, it is essential that you stick to the daily routine and make sure that the baby receives levothyroxine each day. If you are having any problems sticking to treatment, speak to your doctor or nurse as soon as possible.

Children with hypothyroidism

Hypothyroidism can also emerge later in childhood and, as in adults, levothyroxine is the treatment of choice. Children with hypothyroidism usually rapidly catch up their peers in growth and development after starting levothyroxine.

However, the BSPED notes that the personality of some children changes and, not surprisingly, their energy levels rise dramatically once the levothyroxine replaces the missing thyroid hormone. In some cases, their school performance and behaviour may worsen after starting treatment. But be patient: these problems usually settle. Talk to your specialist if you have any concerns; and you might want inform the school.

The BSPED also notes that relatively mild Hashimoto's thyroiditis may settle down as children mature. So they may be able to stop treatment after they stop growing. However, you or your child should never stop or change the dose of a treatment without speaking to your specialist first.

You must make sure your child attends for the blood tests that ensure the dose is correct. These tests generally become less common as the baby gets older. However, the dose of levothyroxine will probably need to increase as the child grows up, to meet his or her changing metabolic demands.

9

Drugs, diseases and the thyroid

As we have seen throughout this book, numerous factors can influence your risk of developing an over- or underactive thyroid gland. This chapter considers the medicines and various other ailments that can trigger or exacerbate thyroid disease.

Drug-induced thyroid problems

As we saw previously (page 14), numerous drugs can influence thyroid function tests. And some medicines can trigger overt thyroid disease in susceptible people. For example certain cough mixtures and supplements contain iodine. So always ensure that your doctor knows which medicines and supplements you are taking, even if you bought the treatment without a prescription. And always tell your pharmacist that you have thyroid disease before buying medicines or collecting a prescription.

Amiodarone

Amiodarone, used to control abnormally fast heartbeats, contains 75 mg of iodine in each 200 mg tablet, which is about 200 times the normal daily iodine requirement.[4] As a result, between 5 and 25 per cent of people taking amiodarone develop hypothyroidism. Hyperthyroidism emerges in between 2 and 10 per cent of amiodarone users. Not surprisingly, the longer you take amiodarone the greater the risk of developing one of these thyroid problems.[6]

Amiodarone-induced hyperthyroidism is most common in areas of the world that are deficient in iodine and in people with Hashimoto's thyroiditis.[6] Furthermore, studies in rats have linked amiodarone to thyroid tumours. Some studies in humans also suggest a possible link between thyrotoxicosis caused by amiodarone and thyroid cancer.[63] However, further studies are needed to fully characterize the risk. So it is important to discuss the risks and benefits with your doctor; there is often an alternative medicine.

Lithium

Lithium is a mood stabilizer used to alleviate bipolar disorder (previously called manic depression) and some other serious mental illnesses. Both the pituitary gland and hypothalamus (page 8) concentrate lithium. A high concentration of lithium inside these critical areas of the brain can interfere with the normal function of the pituitary gland and hypothalamus, including their control of thyroid hormone production (page 7). As a result, depending on the study, between 50 and 100 per cent of people taking lithium show an exaggerated TSH response and reduced secretion of thyroid hormone.[64]

While amiodarone and lithium are the best-known examples, several other drugs can influence thyroid function:

- Opioids (morphine and related potent painkillers), growth hormone and glucocorticoids (a type of steroid used to reduce inflammation) may decrease TSH secretion.[22]
- Glucocorticoids and propranolol (a beta-blocker – see page 10) can suppress the conversion of T_4 to T_3.[16]
- Oral contraceptives or pregnancy can increase levels of the proteins that transport thyroid hormone (as mentioned in Chapter 8).[18]

In addition, several drugs may interfere with the binding of thyroid hormone to the carrier proteins (page 4), including:[16]

- Aspirin and related drugs
- Furosemide: a diuretic ('water tablet') that increases the amount of fluid you excrete (doctors may prescribe diuretics for several diseases, including hypertension and heart failure)
- Heparin: used to prevent blood clots, for example after an operation
- Sulphonylureas: used to treat type 2 diabetes
- Oestrogens (e.g. in HRT and oral contraceptives)
- Glucocorticoids.

This list is not exhaustive and research consistently refines our understanding of a drug's effects. Indeed, uncommon side effects usually emerge only once drugs are on the market and doctors use the medicine in a larger number and more diverse range of patients than included in the clinical studies that drug companies perform to be allowed to sell the drug.

So always check any medicine your doctor suggests you take, using the patient information leaflets included in every pack or the summary of product characteristics (a more detailed summary aimed at health care professionals) here: <www.medicines.org.uk/emc>. These documents warn of interactions between the medicines you are taking. If you have any concerns please speak to your doctor or a pharmacist. Medicine is all about balancing a treatment's risks and benefits, an issue I explore in detail in *The Holistic Health Handbook*.

Illnesses and thyroid disease

Illness can place heavy demands on your body as you fight the disease and marshal your resources to recover. Some infections can spread throughout the body and reach the thyroid. So, not surprisingly, thyroid function is often abnormal in people ill enough to be admitted to hospital:

- Between 2 and 3 per cent of people in hospital show suppressed or elevated blood levels of TSH. However, fewer than half of these have underlying thyroid disorders.[25]
- Only about a quarter of patients admitted to acute care and geriatric hospitals with low blood levels of TSH had hyperthyroidism.[25]
- In another study, 73 per cent of patients aged over 65 years admitted to hospital showed abnormal thyroid tests. Only about 7 per cent had overt or subclinical hypothyroidism. Just over 4 per cent had overt or subclinical hyperthyroidism.[65]

Fortunately, thyroid disease triggered by illness is usually short-lived: for example, T_3 tests return to normal within a month of discharge in 30 per cent of people.[65]

On the other hand, thyroid function tests can predict the risk of death in people aged over 65 years admitted to hospital, even several months after discharge.[65] In one study, for instance, people with low levels of TSH, free T_4 and, in particular, free T_3 on admission to hospital had a worse outlook than those with normal thyroid function. Researchers split patients into three groups based on their free T_3 level. Overall, patients lived for an average of 9 months. However, the average time until death was:

- 3 months in the group with the lowest level of free T_3

- 13 months in the middle group
- 19 months in those with the highest free T_3 level.[65]

People with low levels of free T_3 were also more likely to die from cardiovascular causes. Only about 6 per cent of people with normal free T_3 levels died during hospitalization from cardiovascular disease, compared with 20 per cent of those with low levels.[65] Against this background, it might be prudent to ask your doctor to measure your thyroid function if you have been admitted to hospital and carefully follow his or her instructions following discharge. Just because you have left hospital does not necessarily mean that you are cured.

Viral and bacterial infections

Some viruses and bacteria can infect the thyroid gland. For example, certain bacteria, such as staphylococci and streptococci, can cause boils under the skin. In the thyroid gland, these bacteria can produce large amounts of pus and the inflamed gland becomes very painful. Most people also develop a high fever and the infection may spread to other parts of the body. You may need to have the pus drained or need a course of potent antibiotics.[4]

In other cases, a virus can infect the gland. Viruses use your cellular machinery to replicate and release new viral particles into the body, which allows the infection to spread. According to the British Thyroid Foundation, several viruses can cause thyroiditis, which usually causes an enlarged and painful or tender gland when touched or swallowing. Many people also experience a sore throat, flu-like symptoms and a fever. Viral thyroiditis initially produces symptoms of hyperthyroidism (page 50), sometimes followed by hypothyroidism (page 30). The discomfort caused by viral thyroiditis tends to last for weeks or months. Doctors call this pattern 'subacute'. In some cases, however, a virus, such as Coxsackie or mumps virus, does not cause any discomfort in the gland, but the person still develops symptoms (silent thyroiditis).[4]

As usual with thyroid disease, women are more likely than men to develop viral thyroiditis, which is most common between the ages of 20 and 50 years. Usually, doctors diagnose viral thyroiditis based on signs, symptoms and blood tests. A radioiodine scan (page 19) can rule out other causes of hyperthyroidism, especially if the problem persists.

Viral thyroiditis may improve rapidly without treatment – and so never come to a doctor's attention – or with the help of aspirin or other anti-inflammatory drugs. According to the British Thyroid Foundation, most people recover in 2–5 months. However, about 1 in 20 people with viral thyroiditis develop permanent hypothyroidism. Taking steroids, which reduce inflammation, for 1–2 months usually alleviates persistent pain and other symptoms. The short course limits steroid-related side effects.

Hepatitis C and thyroid disease

Reports of jaundice (yellow skin and eyes caused by the build-up of toxic chemicals produced by the body) that spreads between people date back to ancient Greece. Today, we know that five viruses – hepatitis A to E – are among the most common causes of liver disease. All five viruses replicate inside, and so damage, liver cells.

As the body tries to eradicate the virus, the immune system targets the infected liver cells, which can cause swelling, inflammation (hepatitis), heavy scarring (cirrhosis) and, eventually, liver cancer. Indeed, viral hepatitis causes around a third of new cases of hepatocellular carcinoma, the most common liver cancer, in the UK each year, as discussed in my book *Coping with Liver Disease*.

Hepatitis C virus (HCV), for example spreads, when blood from an infected person gets into another person's bloodstream. Around 93 per cent of the people with chronic (long-standing) HCV in England and Wales contracted the virus through intravenous drug use. You can also catch HCV from blood transfusions and blood products (especially administered aboard), sex, dirty needles (e.g. acupuncture, tattooing and piercing) and transmission from other members of the same household.

Soon after infection with HCV you may experience, for example, fatigue (from mild to severe), poor appetite, weight loss, depression, anxiety, problems with memory and concentration, pain or discomfort in the abdomen. As you can see, these are very similar symptoms to those caused by thyroid disease. This can make the diagnosis difficult. Furthermore, chronic infection with HCV and one of the treatments (called interferon alfa) can cause both hypo- and hyperthyroidism.[66]

In other words, thyroid disease can arise from a multitude of causes. So if your thyroid feels sore or you develop symptoms that could indicate an under- or overactive thyroid, always speak to your doctor.

10

Food and thyroid disease

As mentioned in the Introduction, goitre was, traditionally, common in many mountainous areas. Indeed, healers recognized the intimate link between food and thyroid disease millennia ago. For instance, the Ancient Greeks linked goitre to drinking snow water.[3]

This chapter looks at how your food choices can help you manage your thyroid disease. We will also look at how you can control weight, a common problem for people living with thyroid disease. We will not specifically discuss the basics of healthy eating, which numerous other books cover, including my *Heart Attack Survival Guide* and *The Diabetes Healing Diet*. The British Dietetic Association also publishes an excellent range of fact sheets (including one on iodine) that help you make healthy food choices for you and your family (see 'Useful addresses').

Nevertheless, there is considerable overlap between a healthy diet for people with thyroid disease and a healthy diet generally, so if you are in charge of shopping, the rest of your family will benefit. However, if you radically change your diet, you might influence your levels of thyroid hormone. (Remember that thyroid hormone controls your metabolism.) Therefore let your doctor know: she or he may suggest monitoring your thyroid function and you should watch for any symptoms that might suggest that your thyroid control is changing.

Iodine-rich foods

According to the World Health Organization, most adults need about 150 µg of iodine each day. You can get that much by drinking a pint of milk. Pregnant and breastfeeding women need about 250 µg each day (page 81) to meet the increased demands on their body and keep their baby well supplied with this essential nutrient. However, as we have seen, many pregnant women do not consume enough iodine.

Seaweed

The sea contains most of the world's iodine. So fish (page 99) is a good source of iodine and other nutrients. Seaweed concentrates iodine: levels in kelp are up to 100,000 times greater than in the surrounding water.[67] Seaweed is also packed full of numerous other nutrients, including calcium, phosphorus, magnesium, selenium, manganese and iron. Indeed, seaweed's mineral content is about ten times higher than plants grown in soil and is, generally, a better source of iron than spinach and egg yolks. Seaweed is also high in soluble and insoluble fibre (page 103).[67]

Kelp and other brown seaweeds contain more iodine than the green forms. For instance, *konbu*, a type of kelp, contains 100–1,000 times more iodine than the purple–red seaweed laver, used to make laverbread (laver is called *nori* in Eastern cuisines). The amount of iodine also depends on where the seaweed grew and the processing after harvesting.[67]

However, the British Dietetic Association warns that kelp can provide 'excessive amounts' of iodine. The association recommends eating seaweed no more than once a week. Indeed, adults should, unless advised otherwise by a doctor or dietician, consume no more than 600 µg of iodine each day to avoid triggering thyroid problems. Nevertheless, you could try some Japanese recipes to increase your uptake – cuisine from the Land of the Rising Sun is not all sushi.

Milk and dairy products

Milk and dairy products are another great source of iodine. As cows graze, they concentrate the iodine from the soil and grass in their milk. Ironically, the increasing number of people with thyroid disease could be due, in part, to a 'healthy' diet. A low-salt, non-dairy diet contains relatively little iodine. In addition, organic milk, the British Dietetic Association comments, contains about 40 per cent less iodine than conventional milk. This is because conventional farmers often use weedkillers to control clover, some forms of which can cause goitres in cattle, but organic farmers don't. If you cannot tolerate dairy products, make sure that your soya milk is fortified with iodine.

Milk's importance as a source of iodine underscores the importance of a balanced diet. Focusing excessively on any one part – reducing fat, for example, by avoiding diary food – can cause problems else-

Table 10.1 Guide to the average iodine content of foods

Food	Portion size	Approximate iodine content (micrograms)
White fish	100 g	115
Shellfish	100 g	90
Yoghurt	150 g	50–100
Cow's milk (conventional)	200 ml	50–80
Cow's milk (organic)	200 ml	30–65
Oily fish	100 g	50
Eggs	1 egg/50 g	20
Cheese	40 g	15
Meat	100 g	10
Poultry	100 g	10
Nuts	25 g	5
Bread	1 slice (36 g)	5
Fruit and vegetables	1 portion (80 g)	3

Source: Adapted from the British Dietetic Association

where. You need to eat a healthy, balanced and varied diet. Mary Roach notes that the average person regularly eats no more than about 30 foods. You could keep a note of what you eat for a month. You might be surprised at how limited your choices are.

Table 10 helps you choose foods that help you get enough iodine. However, the amount of iodine in food depends on the soil, farming practice, fish species and so on. Cow's milk and yoghurt tend to contain more iodine during winter, for example. In other words, the figures are rough guides.

Iodine supplements

A balanced diet containing milk, dairy products and fish should mean you get enough iodine. However, vegetarians, and especially vegans, are at high risk of iodine deficiency and could benefit from taking a supplement containing the mineral. You might also want to try a supplement if you feel a bit low, your hair or skin seem dry or you have other *mild* symptoms of iodine deficiency – assuming, of course, you have not been diagnosed with thyroid disease or experience severe symptoms, in which case see your doctor. As we have seen, a supplement can boost your consumption during pregnancy or while breastfeeding (page 82). And some people simply do not like dairy foods or fish: they would prefer a kelp, seaweed and iodine supplement.

Be careful not to consume more than 600 µg of iodine each day from your food, drink and supplements. In addition, the British Dietetic Association warns, levels of iodine in some supplements can vary from that on the label. So take potassium iodide and do not exceed 150 µg of iodine each day from the supplement, unless you are pregnant, breastfeeding or your doctor advises you otherwise. In addition, iron, selenium, manganese and zinc are essential for normal thyroid function.[2] So check that the supplement contains these essential minerals (page 106).

Salt and iodine

In some parts of the world, governments make fortifying salt (sodium chloride) with iodine compulsory. The UK does not, as changes in dairy farming after the 1930s increased milk's iodine content.[10] However, you can buy iodized salt from some health food shops and supermarkets. Nevertheless, excessive salt is bad for your health. So do not rely on iodized salt alone.

For example, we have seen that blood pressure increases to dangerously high levels (hypertension) in about 30 per cent of people with hypothyroidism.[6] High levels of salt in your blood can damage your cells. As a result, your body retains fluid to dilute the salt. This, in turn, increases blood pressure. In other words, a high salt intake makes hypertension more likely. Moreover, the World Cancer Research Fund estimates that excessive salt causes around 1 in 7 stomach cancers.

Unfortunately, almost everyone in the UK eats too much salt. According to the NHS, the average adult eats around 8.1 g of salt a day – about 2 teaspoons. The recommended intake for healthy adults is 6 g of salt a day. But follow your doctor's advice: some people – for example, if you also have liver disease, heart failure or hypertension – need to eat even less.

It is easy to tell that some snacks, such as crisps and salted peanuts, contain large amounts of salt. However, sometimes your taste buds do not set alarm bells ringing. For example, manufacturers add surprisingly large amounts of salt to some soups, bread, biscuits and breakfast cereals. Indeed, salt already added to food during manufacture accounts for 75–80 per cent of our daily consumption.

Fortunately, reducing salt is relatively straightforward: Norwegian researchers found that manufacturers could reduce the amount of salt by between 25 and 30 per cent in some processed foods without changing the taste. To cut your salt intake:

- Avoid foods (such as smoked meat and fish) that are high in salt.
- Add as little salt as you can during baking and cooking.
- Banish the salt-cellar from the table.
- Ask restaurants and takeaways for no salt.
- Look for low-salt ketchup, pickles, mustard, yeast extract, stock cubes and so on.
- Try using herbs, spices, chopped chillies and lime or lemon juice to give grains and other blander foods more taste.

The British Dietetic Association advises choosing meals and sandwiches with less than 0.5 g sodium (1.25 g salt) per meal. Choose individual foods, such as soups and sauces, with less than 0.3 g sodium (0.75 g) per serving. Some labels list sodium rather than salt. To convert sodium to salt, multiply by 2.5. So 0.4 g of sodium is 1 g of salt. You can convert salt to sodium by dividing by 2.5 (see Table 10.2).

Table 10.2 Salt levels in food

Level	Salt content (g in 100 g)	Sodium content (g in 100 g)
High	More than 1.5	More than 0.6
Medium	0.3 to 1.5	0.1 to 0.6
Low	0.3 or less	0.1 or less

Source: Adapted from the British Dietetic Association

Fish and the thyroid

Life inside the Arctic Circle is tough. Few plants survive and the traditional diet of First Nations Arctic people consists of fish and animals that eat marine life, such as seals. Despite their meat-based diet, First Nations Arctic people seem to be less vulnerable to numerous conditions – including diabetes, heart disease, arthritis and asthma – than people in industrialized countries. As this illustrates, eating fish is an important part of a healthy, balanced diet.

As the sea contains most of the world's iodine, seafood, fish and animals that eat fish are a great source of this essential mineral. Fish are also rich in omega-3 fatty acids, also called omega-3 polyunsaturated fatty acids (PUFA), which seem to account for much of the health benefits offered by the Arctic diet. A list of fish and seafood high in omega-3 fatty acids is given in Table 10.3. For example, eating fish once or twice a week (30–60 g per day) reduces the risk of deaths from heart disease by between 30 and 60 per cent.[68] So fish can help bolster a heart-healthy lifestyle if your thyroid disease has driven up your cardiovascular risk.

In addition, oily fish – such as salmon, mackerel and herring – the British Dietetic Association points out, keep joints healthy, while omega-3 PUFAs are important for memory, intellectual performance and healthy vision. Again, we have seen that thyroid disease can impair cognitive performance, and eye problems are common. Although there is little direct evidence for the benefit of fish in thyroid disease, following the dietary advice about fish won't hurt. After all, your mother was right: fish really is brain food.

Table 10.3 Fish and seafood high in omega-3 fatty acids

Anchovy
Black cod (sablefish)
Crab
Dogfish (rock salmon)
Halibut
Herring
Mackerel
Mussels
Oysters
Pilchards
Rainbow trout
Sardines
Salmon
Tuna

Source: Adapted from the University of Michigan and the British Dietetic Association

The British Dietetic Association advises that adults and children over 12 years of age should eat two portions of fish per week. (A portion is about 140 g once cooked). One of these meals should be an oily fish. Omega-3 PUFA levels are higher in fresh fish. If you eat canned fish, check the label to make sure processing has not depleted the omega-3 oils. I believe that it is worth trying to check that the fish comes from sustainable stocks at <www.fishonline. org>.

If at first you do not like the taste, do not give up without trying some different fish and a few recipes. There are plenty of suggest-ions on the internet (e.g. <www.thefishsociety.co.uk>) and in cookbooks. For an island nation, our tastes in fish are remarkably conservative.

If you really cannot stomach the taste of oily fish, you could try a supplement. As usual, speak to your doctor first. For example, if you have diabetes, you may need to avoid omega-3 supplements, which may increase blood sugar levels.

A low-fat diet

Despite its bad press, cholesterol is essential for health and well-being. Cholesterol is a building block of the membranes around every cell. Cholesterol helps form the sheath that surrounds many nerves that ensures signals travel properly. And cholesterol forms the backbone of several hormones, including the sex hormones oestrogen, testosterone and progesterone.

However, poor diets and a lack of exercise (which burns fat) mean that many of us have too much of a good thing. Indeed, 8 million people in the UK regularly take statins – drugs that lower levels of fats in the blood.[69] In any case, medicines do not replace a healthy, low-fat diet. Doctors should prescribe lipid-lowering drugs only if diet alone does not work. Moreover, to gain the most benefit you need to keep eating a healthy diet.

Risks of statins

Lipid-lowering drugs, such as statins, can reduce your risk of a heart attack or stroke. However, like any medicine, statins can cause side effects, including muscle pain, diabetes, liver and kidney problems, cataracts, sexual problems, decreased energy, excessive fatigue and psychiatric symptoms.[70] For example, one study included 10,138 people taking, or who had used, statins. Of these, 29 per cent reported experiencing new or worse muscle pain while taking a statin. About 15 per cent had stopped taking a statin because of muscle pain at least once.[71]

Unfortunately, some side effects of statins – including sexual problems, decreased energy, excessive fatigue and psychiatric changes – overlap with the symptoms of thyroid disease. As a result, doctors should properly investigate the cause. For example, if you stop the statin (under your doctor's supervision of course) and the symptoms abate then recur when you take the lipid-lowerer again, the drugs rather than your thyroid may be responsible. If symptoms persist when you stop the statin, thyroid disease could be to blame. You might find that changing statins resolves the problem.

Furthermore, some other drugs can interact with statins to increase the risk of muscle pain, including certain antibiotics and some medicines for cardiovascular disease, cancer, psychiatric conditions and HIV. So it is prudent to check with your doctor or pharmacist and also to check the patient information leaflet and summary of product characteristics (page 92).

Countering cholesterol confusion

The amount of cholesterol circulating around your body in your blood depends more on how much saturated (animal) fat you eat than the cholesterol in your diet. Indeed, few foods – with the exception of eggs, kidneys, prawns and liver – contain high levels of cholesterol. As a result, cholesterol in our diet accounts for only around a third of the cholesterol in our bodies.

Eggs, for example, are highly nutritious, which makes sense when you think how well they support growth. Eggs are rich in protein, vitamins A, B, D and E, zinc, iron and other minerals. It is fine to go to work on an egg (ideally, boiled or poached rather than fried) as part of a balanced diet.

Rather than worrying about cholesterol, focus on saturated fat, which the liver converts into cholesterol. The British Dietetic Association notes that most people in the UK eat about 20 per cent more than the recommended amount: no more than 20 g and 30 g of saturated fat a day for women and men, respectively. So:

- Eat more low-fat foods, which contain 1.5 g or less saturated fat in 100 g.
- Eat fewer high-fat foods, which contain more than 5 g of saturated fat in 100 g.

Fibre and your bowels

Thyroid disease often changes your bowel habit, causing constipation and diarrhoea. Eating enough fibre can help improve your bowel habit and reduce cardiovascular risk linked to thyroid disease. Indeed, regularly eating whole grains as part of a low-fat diet cuts the risk of heart disease by up to 30 per cent.[25] These studies were not performed specifically in people with thyroid disease, although there is no reason why you would not benefit. If anything, the benefit might be greater because you are at higher risk.

Dietary fibre is the part of plants that we cannot digest, such as the outer layers of sweetcorn, beans, wheat and corn. There are two main types:

- Insoluble fibre remains largely intact as it moves through your digestive system, and makes defecation easier.
- Soluble fibre dissolves in water in the gut, forming a gel that soaks up fats. So you absorb less fat from a meal, which lowers your cholesterol levels. Soluble fibre also releases sugar slowly, which helps stave off hunger pangs and helps you lose weight.

Whole grains are an especially rich source of fibre. Grains – the seeds of cereals, such as wheat, rye, barley, oats and rice – have three parts:

- Bran, the outer layer, is rich in fibre and packed with nutrients. Bran covers the germ and endosperm.
- The nutrient-packed germ develops into a new plant. Wheatgerm, for example, contains high levels of vitamin E, folate (folic acid), zinc, magnesium and other vitamins and minerals.

- The central area (endosperm) is high in starch and provides the energy the germ needs to develop into a new plant.

Food manufacturers often refine grain by stripping off the bran and germ, keeping the white endosperm. However, whole grains contain up to 75 per cent more nutrients than refined cereals, the British Dietetic Association points out.

So it's important to eat enough fibre. Indeed, everyone should, dieticians recommend, eat at least 18 g of fibre each day. Currently, women and men in the UK eat on average only 13 g and 15 g, respectively. Furthermore, 95 per cent of adults in the UK do not eat enough whole grains. About a third do not eat any. The British Dietetic Association advocates getting at least half your starchy carbohydrates from whole grains (two to three servings daily). Try eating more foods with 'whole' in front of the name, such as whole-wheat pasta and whole oats.

Fibre and irritable bowel syndrome

As we have mentioned (page 35), doctors may mistakenly diagnose IBS instead of thyroid disease. You might also develop IBS by coincidence or because you are stressed with your thyroid condition or life in general. IBS is one of those diseases that is strongly influenced by your mental state.

Dietary and lifestyle advice is the foundation of IBS management. However, insoluble fibre may exacerbate pain and distension if you suffer from constipation as part of your IBS or thyroid disease. So introduce fibre gradually into your diet.[72] You could also try soluble fibre such as ispaghula powder (speak to your doctor or pharmacist) or foods high in soluble fibre (e.g. oats).[73] According to the British Society for Gastroenterology, some people find that dairy products, onions, nuts and drinks containing caffeine (e.g. coffee, tea and cola) exacerbate IBS. You could try eliminating these from your diet. But do not eliminate important foods (such as bread and other gluten-containing foods or dairy products) unless you are being supervised by a doctor or, ideally, a dietician.

Your doctor can prescribe several drugs for IBS to help control the most troublesome symptoms, such as constipation, pain or bloating.[72] Several complementary treatments – including cognitive behavioural therapy (CBT), hypnotherapy and active relaxation – may also help. Chapter 11 includes more about these approaches.

Five portions of fruit and vegetables

Fruit and vegetables are a great source of fibre and other nutrients. In general, fruits and vegetables do not contain much iodine. But as we saw in Chapter 3, certain foods, including cruciferous vegetables (such as cabbage, cauliflower, broccoli and turnips), can contribute to goitres.[2] Langer and Scheer report (see 'Further reading') that some European communities facing famine during the First World War survived by eating large amounts of cabbage and turnips. Most developed goitres. Kale and seaweed are staples of Tasmanian and Japanese cuisine, respectively, and are also potential goitrogens.[4]

Today, almost no one eats enough of these to make a difference, especially in parts of the world where there is enough iodine in food and water. Nevertheless, if you have hypothyroidism, Patsy Westcott advises limiting your intake of foods that can reduce iodine uptake, such as Brussels sprouts, broccoli, cabbage, millet, peanuts, pine nuts and turnips.[7]

Nevertheless, you must still eat at least five portions of fruit and vegetables each day. A portion weighs about 80 g, and examples of one portion of fruit or vegetables are given in Table 10.4. Cooking can leach nutrients from fruits and vegetables. So either eat fruit raw or cook vegetables using a small amount of unsalted water for the shortest time you can, or try steaming and stir-frying.

Table 10.4 One portion of fruit of vegetables

One medium-sized fruit (banana, apple, pear, orange)
One slice of a large fruit (melon, pineapple, mango)
Two smaller fruits (plums, satsumas, apricots, peaches)
A dessert bowl full of salad
Three heaped tablespoonfuls of vegetables
Three heaped tablespoons of pulses (chickpeas, lentils, beans)
Two to three tablespoons ('a handful') of grapes or berries
One tablespoon of dried fruit
One glass (150 ml) of unsweetened fruit or vegetable juice or smoothie (if you drink two or more glasses of juice a day, it still only counts as one portion)

Supplements and the thyroid

Supplements can help tackle specific problems arising from an under- or overactive thyroid. However, it is always best to double check with your doctor if you are in any doubt, have been diagnosed with a serious disease or are taking any medicine. And never take more than the recommended amount.

Some drugs can interact with supplements – as we saw with the dosing restrictions around levothyroxine (page 42). Always tell your pharmacist about any supplements you are taking when you collect a prescription or buy a medicine. Stop taking the supplement and see your doctor if you feel unwell.

B Vitamins

According to the British Dietetic Association, low levels of the B vitamins thiamine (B$_1$), niacin (B$_3$) or cobalamin (B$_{12}$) can cause tiredness and leave you feeling depressed or irritable. In other words, low levels of B vitamins could exacerbate some symptoms of thyroid disease. Try to boost your intake of fortified foods (such as cereals), meat, fish and dairy products. Check the label to see whether the food is fortified. Again, you can take supplements to boost your intake.

The British Dietetic Association notes that low levels of folate (folic acid; vitamin B$_9$) can increase the chance that you will feel depressed. Making sure you get enough folate is particularly important as you get older – and thyroid disease becomes more common with advancing age. Liver, green vegetables, oranges and other citrus fruits, beans and fortified foods (such as Marmite and breakfast cereals) are good sources.

Finally, if you are trying to conceive, make sure you get enough folic acid. All women who are planning to have a baby or who are pregnant should take folic acid supplements to reduce the risk of neural tube defects such as spina bifida. If you have any questions, talk to your midwife, GP or health visitor.

Beta-carotene

Beta-carotene is the orange–red pigment that gives carrots, pumpkins, peppers, yams and so on their characteristic colour. In other foods rich in beta-carotene – including spinach, asparagus and broccoli – the green chlorophyll, which converts sunlight into energy, masks the beta-carotene. Thyroid hormone stimulates the liver to convert beta-carotene into vitamin A.[7] It's a good idea to try to eat enough of these vegetables and consider a multivitamin containing beta-carotene. Vitamin A itself, in high doses, can be toxic. So you are better off eating beta-carotene than vitamin A.

Iron

Iron carries oxygen around your body in your blood. So low levels of iron can cause anaemia and leave you feeling weak, tired and lethargic. Once again, depleted iron levels can exacerbate the low energy, weakness and fatigue caused by subclinical or overt hypothyroidism. In addition, the heavy periods experienced by some women with thyroid disease can deplete iron stores. Red meat in particular, as well as poultry and fish, are good sources of iron. (Trim any visible fat away.) If you are a vegetarian, vegan or do not eat much red meat, you may need supplements containing iron.

Magnesium

Magnesium helps your body use calcium, which keeps your bones strong. So getting enough magnesium (as well as calcium) may help reduce the risk of fractures caused by osteoporosis (page 6). Figs, lemons, grapefruit, sweetcorn, almonds, nuts, seeds, dark-green vegetables and apples are rich in magnesium.

Manganese

Manganese – found in nuts, green leafy vegetables, peas, beetroot, egg yolks and wholegrain cereals – is involved in the production of thyroid hormone.[7]

Selenium

Low levels of selenium may increase the chance of feeling depressed. Brazil nuts, meat, fish and bread are good sources of selenium. A supplement may help improve mood in some people who do not get enough selenium from food. As discussed in Chapter 6, selenium supplements may help people with mild thyroid eye disease.

Weight control and thyroid disease

Thyroid hormone controls the amount of energy you release from food, and when you eat more, T_3 levels rise. When you diet, your metabolism decreases and T_3 levels fall. This reduced rate of metabolism helps protect us from starvation. The same mechanism means that people with anorexia, bulimia or even those who diet excessively often develop 'sluggish' thyroids.[7]

As this suggests, thyroid diseases can affect your appetite and weight. If you have had hyperthyroidism, the increased activity helped keep your weight down. So when treatment resolves the thyroid problem, you may find you gain weight. Once you are at your ideal weight, you may need to modify your diet to keep your weight under control.

If you have an underactive thyroid gland you may gain a few pounds. For example, tiredness, lack of energy, joint and muscle pains and stiffness can lead to inactivity, Martin Budd remarks. You may crave sugar to give yourself a boost. Depression can also sap your will to stay active. Indeed, Budd found that many people, even with relatively mild hypothyroidism, often find it difficult to lose weight and keep it off. You will probably stop gaining weight when treatment restores normal thyroid hormone levels, but you will need to exercise and diet to lose any weight you have gained.

Unfortunately, losing weight is not easy – whatever the latest fad diets would have you believe. After all, millions of years of evolution drive us to consume food in times of feast to help us survive times of famine. And you cannot stop eating as you can quit smoking or drinking alcohol. However, the following tips may help:

- Keep a food diary and record everything you eat and drink for a couple of weeks. It is often easy to see where you inadvertently pile on the extra calories: the odd biscuit here, the extra glass of wine or full-fat latte there. It soon adds up. A food diary can also help you see if you are eating fatty or high-salt food.
- Set a realistic, specific target. Rather than saying that you want to lose weight, resolve to lose a certain amount, such as 10 kg or 2 stones. Calculate your body mass index (BMI) – the easiest way is to use an online calculator – to set your target. Cutting your intake by between 500 and 1,000 calories each day can reduce bodyweight (assuming your BMI is stable) by between 0.5 and

1.0 kg (1–2 lb) each week. Steadily losing around a pound or two each week makes it less likely you will put it on again.

- Think about how you tried to lose weight in the past. What techniques and diets worked? Which failed to make a difference or proved impossible to stick to? Did going to a support group help?
- Do not let a slip-up derail your diet. Try to identify why you indulged. What were the triggers? Was it a particular occasion? Do you comfort eat? Once you know why you slipped you can develop strategies to stop another slip-up.
- Begin your diet when you are at home over a weekend or a holiday and you do not have a celebration (such as Christmas or a birthday) planned. It is tougher changing your diet on a Monday morning or when you are away on business in a hotel faced with fat-laden food, caffeine-rich drinks and alcohol.

If this fails, talk to your GP or pharmacist. Several medicines may help kick-start your weight loss. You can also try cognitive behavioural therapy (CBT; see page 122) and hypnosis. CBT can reduce weight by 2.75 kg (around 6 lb). Adding hypnosis (page 118) to CBT can increase weight loss to 6.75 kg (almost 15 lb).[51]

Changing your diet can seem daunting. But many people find that it takes only a month or so of eating, or not eating, a food for the change to become a habit. For instance, some people (myself among them) who swap full-fat for skimmed milk soon find that they dislike the taste of full-fat milk, which will help keep your iodine intake up without extra calories. Likewise, many people soon lose their sweet tooth or taste for salt.

11

Living well with thyroid disease

Thyroid hormone increases the amount of energy that almost every tissue and organ uses.[6] And your brain is no exception. Indeed, doctors discovered decades ago that thyroid disease can affect your mental state and vice versa. In 1888, for example, the Clinical Society of London heard that patients with myxoedema (page 6) often experienced mental issues, including irritability, agoraphobia (a type of anxiety), dementia and depression.[64]

Stress – such as bereavement, redundancy, divorce, an accident or conflict – increases the risk of developing Graves' disease or suffering an exacerbation. For example, in Serbia, the number of cases of Graves' disease has been broadly stable since 1971. However, the number of people with the disease increased markedly during the 1992–1995 war.[40] Likewise, the number of people with hyperthyroidism in Norway and Denmark rose during the first few years of the Second World War. The number of people with Graves' disease also increased in Northern Ireland during the troubles.[7] These are extreme examples, but it is sensible to try to keep your stress in check.

In addition, a change in appearance caused by thyroid disease – such as thyroid orbitopathy, lacklustre or thinning hair (page 115) or the 'Queen Anne' sign, a thinning or loss of the outer third of the eyebrows – can cause anger, undermine your self-esteem or confidence, contribute to social isolation and even trigger depression.

Once you start treatment, fluctuating thyroid hormone levels can leave you feeling anxious, irritable and prone to mood swings. So your family and friends may need to be sympathetic until your hormone levels stabilize. Taking your medicines as agreed with your doctor can help avoid fluctuating levels. However, some people find the anxiety persists, albeit less intensely, in which case a beta-blocker (page 10) may help.[4] You can also try some of the relaxation techniques in this chapter, while counselling can help you come to terms with living with a chronic condition. In this chapter, we will look at steps you can take to tackle the mental burden imposed by living with thyroid disease.

Thyroid disease and depression

Depression is more than feeling 'a bit down', more than 'the blues': it is a profound, debilitating mental and physical lethargy; a devastating loss of self-esteem; and intense, deep, unshakable sadness. If you have never experienced true (clinical) depression, you cannot appreciate just how dreadful the condition is.

Thyroid disease can directly and indirectly cause or exacerbate depression. The brain controls the amount of thyroid hormone it receives from the blood, using a special 'transport' protein. If this transport system is not working properly, the brain may not get enough thyroid hormone, despite normal levels in the blood. This may contribute to some cases of depression.[64]

Thyroxine and depression

During the early twentieth century, psychiatrists tried a wide range of agents to alleviate depression, including chloral hydrate (the main component of a Mickey Finn), barbiturates, amphetamines and, for agitated people, opiates. They also investigated, with varying success, insulin comas, chemical and electrical shocks and 'sleep cures'.[74]

Today's antidepressants – tricyclic antidepressants, monoamine oxidase inhibitors, selective serotonin reuptake inhibitors (SSRIs) and newer agents such as venlafaxine – all raise levels of a group of chemical signals called monoamine neurotransmitters, which carry messages between nerves. However, around 30 per cent of people do not respond adequately to current antidepressants.[74] Unfortunately, because of their limited range of actions, switching antidepressant does not always help, although it is always worth trying. In one study, the proportion of people whose depression resolved when they switched antidepressant declined from 37 per cent with the first antidepressant to 13 per cent with the fourth treatment.[75] As thyroid hormone acts in a different way from conventional antidepressants, doctors sometimes add levothyroxine if conventional drugs do not alleviate the depression.[64]

Distinguishing depression from hypothyroidism

Some clues may help you distinguish depression from hypothyroidism. For example, in hypothyroidism you gain weight despite a lack of appetite and eating relatively small amounts. In depression, your appetite can change: you may comfort eat or just not feel hungry. In other words, weight tends to be more closely linked to the amount you eat in depression compared with hypothyroidism.[7]

Sleep disturbances are common in depression and thyroid disease. People with hypothyroidism sleep more than usual, but still feel tired.[7] By contrast, about 70 per cent of people with depression experience difficulty falling asleep, frequent or early-morning waking and daytime tiredness. Some people even regard their depression as a predominantly sleep, rather than mood, disorder.[76]

Finally, depression and thyroid disease can undermine self-esteem. For instance, feeling 'low' is part of the normal process of grieving. However, bereavement is a severe psychosocial stressor that can trigger depression in vulnerable people. Typically, grief comes in waves and grieving people maintain their self-esteem. Depression, however, produces persistent distress and undermines self-esteem.[77] In addition, thyroid disease does not usually trigger the profound guilt that is one of the most distressing symptoms of depression.[7] Nevertheless, distinguishing hypothyroidism and depression can prove difficult.

Depression often improves once you are treated for hypothyroidism. However, in some cases you may need antidepressants or counselling if the depression persists after the other symptoms of hypothyroidism have improved. You will probably need to take antidepressants for several days, weeks and, sometimes, months before the hopelessness, helplessness and the suicidal feelings certain people endure abate.[78] So stick with treatment. Once again, a diary may help you realize how much you have improved.

Other psychiatric problems

Depression is not the only psychiatric disease linked to thyroid problems. People with bipolar disorder experience marked mood swings from depression to feeling very high and overactive. (Less severe mania is called hypomania.)

The speed of the mood swings varies markedly. Some people experience more than four cycles a year, a pattern doctors call rapidly cycling bipolar disease. Between 70 and 90 per cent of people with rapidly cycling bipolar disease are women. Furthermore, about 25 per cent of people with rapidly cycling bipolar disease show hypothyroidism, compared with 2–5 per cent of people with bipolar disease overall.[64]

In younger people in particular, hyperthyroidism often causes anxiety. Doctors frequently experience problems differentiating anxiety alone from that caused by hyperthyroidism. Often, however, the anxiety abates when the hyperthyroidism improves.[4] If the anxiety does not improve, your doctor may be able to suggest drugs and counselling. Relaxation techniques (discussed later in this chapter) can also help.

Perchance to dream

Sleep is among the most enigmatic, fascinating and fundamental aspects of biology. Yet despite spending around a third of our lives asleep, it arguably remains the least understood of our fundamental biological processes. As we have seen, hyperthyroidism, depression and hypothyroidism often stop you from getting a good night's sleep. Disturbed sleep may even increase the risk of thyroid cancer (page 77). The stress linked to any thyroid disease can also lead to restless nights.

You can take several steps to help you get a good night's sleep:

- Wind down or relax at the end of the day. Do not go to bed while your mind is racing or pondering problems.
- Try not to take your troubles to bed with you. Brooding makes problems seem worse, exacerbates stress, keeps you awake and, because you are tired in the morning, means you are less able to deal with your difficulties. Likewise, try to avoid heavy discussions before bed.
- Do not worry about anything you have forgotten to do. Get up and jot it down (keep a notepad by the bed if you find you do this commonly). This should help you forget about the problem until the morning.
- Go to bed at the same time each night and set your alarm for the same time each morning, even at weekends. This helps re-establish a regular sleep pattern.
- Avoid naps during the day.

- Avoid stimulants, such as caffeine and nicotine, for several hours before bed. Try hot milk or milky drinks instead.
- Do not drink too much fluid (even if non-alcoholic) just before bed as this can mean regular trips to the bathroom.
- Avoid alcohol. A nightcap can help you fall asleep but as blood levels of alcohol fall, sleep becomes more fragmented and lighter. Therefore, you may wake repeatedly later in the night.
- Do not eat a heavy meal before bedtime.
- Regular exercise helps you sleep. However, exercising just before bed can disrupt sleep.
- Use the bed for sex and sleep only. Do not work or watch TV.
- Make the bed and bedroom as comfortable as possible. Invest in a comfortable mattress, with enough bedclothes, and make sure the room is not too hot, too cold or too bright.
- If you cannot sleep, get up and do something else. Watch the TV or read – nothing too stimulating – until you feel tired. Lying there worrying about not sleeping just keeps you awake.

If all this fails, you could discuss taking a sleeping pill ('hypnotic') with your GP. However, these are only for short-term (1–2 weeks or so) use.

Thyroid disease and sex

A sex life that is right for you and your partner helps build and maintain relationships. Unfortunately, thyroid disease can cause problems in the bedroom other than insomnia:

- Hypothyroidism can sap your sex drive; after all, fatigue and depression are hardly conducive to a satisfying sex life.
- Some physical changes resulting from thyroid disease – gaining or losing weight, dry skin, dull hair and so on – can undermine feelings of attractiveness.
- The sex drive of people with hyperthyroidism can rise, and the constant demands can place a burden on the partner.[7]

Indeed, Andrew Russell notes, the impact on sex life 'is often the most distressing aspect of a chronic illness'. Yet fear of embarrassment means that many doctors do not ask about their patients' sex lives. It is up to you to raise the topic.

Unhealthy hair and thyroid disease

In the UK we spend about £1.5 billion a year on haircare products, and numerous adverts emphasize the sex appeal of attractive coiffure. However, hyper- and hypothyroidism can lead to hair loss and unhealthy hair. During the 2013 European Association of Dermatology and Venereology Congress, researchers from Romania reported that 11 per cent of women with female-pattern hair loss had underlying thyroid disease. Unfortunately, hair can take up to 2 years to regrow, despite treating the underlying thyroid disease:[4] hair grows by about 1 cm a month.[79] In the meantime, regular haircuts can help control the appearance of thinning, dry hair – or you can buy a hat.[7]

So try talking to a counsellor or ask your doctor, nurse or patient group what may help give your sex life a boost, such as:

- not drinking too much alcohol;
- creating a relaxing atmosphere;
- getting into a comfortable position;
- asking your partner to take a more active role.

In other cases, some drugs (including some antidepressants and beta-blockers) can affect your sex drive or cause impotence. Swallow any embarrassment and speak to your GP if you think a medicine could be causing your impotence or reduced sex drive. Switching treatment may resolve the problem. In addition, GPs and some pharmacists can offer Viagra (sildenafil) and a growing range of other effective treatments for male impotence (properly called erectile dysfunction). But never buy any drug over the internet, unless you are sure the online pharmacy is reputable.

A romantic mood, effectively treating the underlying condition and tackling any issues can help reinvigorate a sex life that stalls in the wake of a thyroid disorder or another serious disease.

Benefits of a strong relationship

A fulfilling sex life helps build a strong relationship. And, as I explored in *The Holistic Health Handbook*, a strong relationship – exemplified by marriage – is valuable for health. (For the sake of brevity, 'married' encompasses other long-term, mutually supportive, cohabiting relationships with a 'significant other'.)

For example, assuming that everything else remains the same, 90 per cent of married 48-year-old women are still alive at 65 years of age compared with 80 per cent of those who never married. Men benefit even more: 90 per cent of married 48-year-old men are still alive at 65 years of age, compared with just 60 per cent of lifelong bachelors.[80] Another study followed 4,802 people aged 40 for 22 years. Those who remained single were twice as likely to die prematurely as those who were consistently married, after allowing for personality and other risk factors. Those who went through the trauma of divorce were 64 per cent more likely to die prematurely.[81]

Not surprisingly, given their increased longevity, married people are less likely to have chronic illness, disability or physical problems than those who remain single. The difference is especially marked when behaviour or lifestyle makes a particular contribution to the illnesses.[80]

In some ways, the suggestion that a strong marriage and other social support networks help bolster your health is not surprising. Close family and friends, and a strong marriage, can give powerful reasons to live as well as offering social, practical and emotional support to help cope with the stress of living with thyroid disease or another chronic ailment. Indeed, people with strong social connections show less marked changes in their blood pressure when they face high levels of negative emotions.[82] A spouse and friends can also give you a nudge to see a doctor when you feel unwell, which may be one reason why married individuals appear more likely to present at the earlier stages of a malignancy.[83] So remind your partner with thyroid disease to make a doctor's appointment if you notice any change in their appearance.

Furthermore, your partner's and family's practical and emotional support can be invaluable if you are trying to drink less alcohol, quit smoking, take more exercise, change your diet and take your medicines as prescribed. For example, your partner can:

- help you adopt a healthy lifestyle;
- ignore bad moods triggered by the disease or when treatment begins;
- boost your motivation to stick with a healthy lifestyle or treatment when you feel like quitting;
- watch for harmful behaviours, such as offering a gentle reminder if you start eating unhealthy food regularly.

However, partners need to tread the fine line between nagging and support. Studies report that a spouse's *support* – helping and reinforcing the efforts of the partner (who had heart disease) to tackle unhealthy behaviours – improved mental health. However, *control* – trying to persuade a partner to adopt healthy behaviours when he or she is unwilling or unable – reduced the likelihood that the spouse would make the changes, and undermined mental health.[84] Indeed, an experimental minor wound healed 40 per cent more slowly in those with 'hostile' marriages.[85] This underscores the potent biological effects produced by relationships.

Exercise

Many people with hypothyroidism find that getting enough exercise is tough. However, exercise increases mobility, strength and stamina. It protects against osteoporosis, hypertension, heart attacks and strokes, and helps you maintain your ideal weight, which is often difficult for people with thyroid disease, even after treatment begins.

Doctors recommend that you should be moderately active for at least 30 minutes on at least 5 days each week – and ideally every day. It does not all have to be in one go. You can exercise for 15 minutes twice a day, for example. Aim to exercise until you are breathing harder than usual, but not so hard that you cannot hold a conversation. You should feel that your heart is beating faster than usual and you have begun to sweat. However, if you experience chest pain, feel faint or otherwise unwell, stop exercising and see your doctor.

Exercise as part of everyday life

Try and make exercise part of everyday life. You lose about half the cardiovascular fitness you have gained after exercising regularly for a year in just 3 months if you stop. So find a type of exercise that you enjoy and that fits into your lifestyle. If you do not like exercise classes and you join a gym some distance from home or work, you are more likely to quit. On the other hand, you can easily integrate walking into your daily life. A pedometer helps ensure you walk at least 10,000 steps every day, as recommended by the American Heart Association.

There are plenty of other opportunities make exercise part of your day-to-day life:

- Walk to the local shops instead of taking the car.
- Ride a bike to work instead of travelling by car or public transport.
- Park a 15-minute walk from your place of work.
- If you take the bus, tube or metro, get off one or two stops early.
- Use the stairs instead of the lift.
- Clean the house regularly and wash your car by hand.
- Grow your own vegetables – and they taste better.

Back to nature

And get out of town. Strolling around country parks and nature reserves brings other benefits than just improving fitness, including enhancing relaxation and boosting the body's ability to treat itself. Indeed, patients who had a view of a natural setting recovered from surgery more rapidly than a similar group who faced a wall.[86] Likewise, Japanese people with chronic illness often benefit from walking in woods – called *shinrin-yoku* (forest bathing) – which, among other benefits, encourages relaxation, reduces stress, lowers blood pressure and boosts the immune system. Even looking at, for example, a picture of people walking in a forest reduced blood pressure. But the smell and other sensations of walking through a forest augment the visual appreciation of natural beauty.[87]

So make the most of the more than 400 country parks and many other nature reserves in England alone. The following are good places to start:

- Natural England: <www.naturalengland.org.uk/ourwork/enjoying/ places/countryparks/countryparksnetwork/findacountrypark>
- The National Trust: <www.nationaltrust.org.uk>
- The Ramblers: <www.ramblers.org.uk/go-walking.aspx>
- The Royal Society for the Protection of Birds: <www.rspb.org.uk/ reserves>
- The Woodland Trust: <visitwoods.org.uk>.

Hypnosis

For centuries, conventional doctors dismissed hypnotism as a stage trick, its benefits confined to weak-willed, gullible people.

In 1890, the *British Medical Journal* called hypnotism 'a dangerous mental poison, and as such it needs to be fenced round with as many restrictions as the traffic in other kinds of poison'. The journal added that hypnotism is 'fraught with many dangers to the nervous equilibrium and psychological soundness of the subject'.[88]

Some doctors even suggested that subjects faked trances to please their hypnotist. Yet Roberta Bivins recounts (see 'Further reading') how in 1842 a 'respectable' surgeon from Nottingham who used hypnotism on the patient while amputating his leg. At the time, alcohol offered the only anaesthetic and patients, not surprisingly, often needed to be drunk and tied down to allow the surgeon to operate. Around the same time, James Esdaile, a Scottish surgeon working near Calcutta, removed a scrotal tumour using hypnosis as anaesthesia. In 1829, the French doctor Pierre-Jean Chapelain used hypnosis as an anaesthetic during a mastectomy for breast cancer.[51] It is hard to believe that someone would endure the pain of a scrotal operation, amputation or mastectomy to please the surgeon. The advent of powerful painkillers and anaesthetics meant that healers no longer resorted to hypnosis, but these examples underscore hypnotism's power.

Today, doctors still do not fully understand how hypnotism works. Essentially, however, hypnosis is focused attention and concentration. Some hypnotists describe the process as similar to being 'so lost in a book or movie that it is easy to lose track of what is going on around you'.[51] And despite the cynicism of Victorian doctors (who probably worried that hypnotism could take some of their business), hypnosis helps with pain, stress and changing harmful habits such as abusing alcohol, comfort eating and smoking.[51]

Hypnosis is safe. You will not lose control, hypnotists cannot make you do or say anything they choose and you can come out of a hypnotic trance whenever you want.[51] Some people also find that self-hypnosis helps them relax and deal with unhealthy behaviours. Numerous DVDs, CDs and books help you create the focused attention that underpins hypnosis. Contact the British Association of Medical Hypnosis for further information.

T'ai chi

Meditation is not confined to sitting in the lotus position chanting 'om'. T'ai chi, yoga and rosary prayer are all forms of meditation and excellent ways to relax. However, learning classical medita-tion can be difficult without guidance. Many local adult education centres hold courses. Your vicar or spiritual adviser can educate you about the best way to pray.

T'ai chi (t'ai chi ch'uan) is a 'soft' or 'internal' martial art that combines deep breathing, meditation and relaxation with sequences (called forms) of slow, gentle movements that enhance fitness, strength and flexibility. This means that t'ai chi is often suitable (after checking with your doctor) for people with thyroid disease or other chronic conditions. Furthermore, if you find exercise difficult, t'ai chi can offer a gentle way to start being more active.

You can learn the t'ai chi short form in about 12 lessons. However, t'ai chi takes many years to master. Speeded up, t'ai chi can offer effective self-defence – indeed, ch'uan means fist. Speed up a raising hand and you may deflect a blow to the head, and a descending hand can deflect a kick. Contact the T'ai Chi Union for Great Britain for more information.

Yoga

Yoga brings millions of people – from all religious backgrounds – inner peace, relief from stress and improved health. Yoga aims to harmonize consciousness, mind, energy and body. (The Indian root of the word yoga means to unite.)

Essentially, yoga focuses on achieving controlled, slow, deep breaths, while the poses (asanas) increase fitness, strength and flexibility. As a result, yoga helps keep your body and mind supple (some of the poses require considerable concentration).

Relatively few studies have assessed yoga in thyroid disease. However, yoga added to conventional treatment seems to improve lung function and the quality of life in people with hypothy-roidism.[89,90] Other studies suggest that yoga may also help people with other diseases linked to thyroid diseases, including anxiety and depression.[91,92] Indeed, yoga improves mood and reduces anxiety more than the same time spent exercising by walking.[93] Contact the British Wheel of Yoga for more information.

> *Think about your breathing*
>
> One of the first things a yoga, martial arts or meditation teacher will probably tell you is that you are not breathing correctly. Most of us breathe shallowly using the upper parts of our lungs. Try putting one hand on your chest and the other on your abdomen. Then breathe normally. Most people find that the hand on their chest moves while the one on the abdomen remains relatively still. To fill your lungs fully, make the hand on your abdomen rise, while keeping the one on the chest as still as possible. Breathing deeply and slowly without gasping helps relaxation. If you feel stressed out, try breathing in deeply through your nose for the count of four, hold your breath for a count of seven and then breathe out for a count of eight. Repeat a dozen times.

Active relaxation

There is nothing wrong with curling up with a good book or watching your favourite television programme. However, many of us need to take a more active approach to relaxation. So, for example, the National Institute for Health and Care Excellence (NICE) notes that relaxation therapies – including progressive muscle relaxation, meditation, yoga, assertiveness training and anger control techniques – reduce blood pressure by around 3.5 mmHg. A third of people using these techniques show at least a 10 mmHg reduction in blood pressure. That's similar to the improvement produced by many drugs for hypertension. However, as usual, do not reduce the dose of any medication or stop therapy without talking to your doctor.

Finding time to relax

The link between mind and body means that you cannot be mentally tense while your body is relaxed or vice versa. Relaxing your body relaxes your mind.

The following tips should help you relax. You may need to adapt these if, for example, you want to meditate or practice yoga.

- Try to follow your relaxation therapy every day. Many people find that the early morning is best for active relaxation. The house is quiet and you will be better able to focus and less likely to drop off to sleep than later at night.

- Make yourself comfortable. Sit in a comfortable chair that supports your back or lie down. You might want to put cushions under your neck and knees. Take off your shoes, switch off any bright lights and ensure the room is neither too hot nor too cold.
- Do not perform relaxation therapy on a full stomach. After a meal, blood diverts from your muscles to your stomach. Trying progressive muscle relaxation (see the next section) on a full stomach can cause cramps. As relaxation can make you more aware of your body's functions, a full stomach can be a distraction.
- Shut your eyes and, if it helps, play some relaxing music and burn some aromatherapy oils. One study, for example, found that the aroma of sweet orange reduces anxiety.[94]

Progressive muscular relaxation

Progressive muscular relaxation (PMR) aims to relax each part of your body in turn. To try PMR, put your hands by your side. Now clench your fists as hard as you can. Hold the fist for 10 seconds. Now slowly relax your fist and let your hands hang loosely by your sides. Then shrug your shoulders as high as you can. Hold for 10 seconds and then relax slowly. Then gently arch your back, hold for 10 seconds and relax. Tense your muscles as you inhale. Do not hold your breath. Try to breathe slowly and rhythmically. Exhale as you relax. Repeat each exercise three times, slowly, gently and gradually. Remember, you are not body building, you are relaxing. Most PMR teachers advise mastering one muscle group at a time; it can take 2–3 months before you can tense and relax your entire body.

We become used to a certain amount of muscle tension. Our neck feels stiff. Our jaw muscles clench. We frown. However, with practice, you will start recognizing when your muscles are tense during your everyday life – and you can then use PMR to relax the tense muscles. However, if you have back problems, arthritis or any other serious disease, check with your doctor before trying PMR.

Counselling and cognitive behavioural therapy (CBT)

Sharing problems, asking for advice or considering a different perspective often helps you overcome problems arising from thyroid disease, another chronic condition or from life generally. Counselling, or contact with other people who have thyroid disease, can help you find coping strategies. So contact the British Thyroid Foundation, the Thyroid Eye Disease Charitable Trust or your local eye centre or thyroid centre for help in locating a support group. Your GP may also be able to suggest a counsellor. But it is worth checking that the counsellor is familiar with the issues facing people with thyroid disease.

Counsellors and psychotherapists use a variety of 'talking therapies' to help you tackle your problems. One widely used approach, CBT, identifies the feelings, thoughts and behaviours associated with thyroid disease or an unhealthy lifestyle. You will question and test those feelings, thoughts, behaviours and beliefs, then learn to replace unhelpful and unrealistic behaviours with approaches that actively address problems. CBT usually uses explicit goals, often broken into manageable, short-term goals and supported by regular 'homework'.

Mindfulness

In some cases, therapists combine CBT with other approaches, such as mindfulness.[95] Essentially, mindfulness encourages you to concentrate, non-judgementally and openly, on the present rather than worry about what might happen or ruminate on the past. Some therapists compare mindfulness to waking up from life on automatic pilot. Mindfulness seems to increase your ability to regulate and manage behaviour as well as improve your flexibility of thinking, emotions and behaviour. As a result, you can adapt more effectively[96] and find new ways to cope with thyroid disease or other problems.

For example, a stress-reduction programme that encompasses mindfulness typically lasts between 8 and 10 weeks and may use meditation and yoga to recognize and escape from habitual, counterproductive thoughts and behaviours. So, used alongside CBT, mindfulness stress reduction helps you accept and tolerate the unpleasant emotions that the therapy or the changing of habitual behaviours may evoke.[96]

Mindfulness-based interventions can alleviate a variety of ailments, including some of those linked to thyroid disease, such as chronic pain, anxiety and depression. Indeed, mindfulness-based CBT may reduce the risk that depression will relapse as effectively as antidepressants, in some people at least.[96] For instance, a study of 469 adults in the UK found that 46 per cent of those who also underwent CBT reported at least a 50 per cent reduction in depression after 6 months, despite showing a poor response to antidepressants alone. This compared with 22 per cent of those managed with 'usual care', such as changing antidepressants or referring to psychiatric services.[97]

To discuss whether CBT or one of the other talking therapies could help you, contact the British Association for Counselling and Psychotherapy or ask your doctor's surgery to recommend a local counsellor.

Complementary therapy and holistic health

If you want to try complementary therapy to help you cope with thyroid disease, check with your doctor first. Then ensure that you consult a registered practitioner, such as one recognized by the General Regulatory Council for Complementary Therapies or the Complementary and Natural Healthcare Council (see 'Useful addresses'). Read up on the approach you are planning to use and make sure you understand the risks and benefits.

Keep a watch for side effects. Some alternative healers believe that complementary therapies drive out toxins that have accumulated in your body. This toxic 'tsunami' can produce a detox 'crisis', characterized by unpleasant symptoms such as headaches, fatigue and abdominal discomfort. In some cases, the healer and the person undergoing detox can dismiss adverse events as a crisis. So you need to be careful if you experience any unexpected symptoms.

You need to check the treatments work. As mentioned before, one of the best ways is to keep a diary noting the symptoms, triggers and how you feel. If you do not feel any benefit after 3 months, consider whether it is worth continuing.

Try to keep optimistic

Healthy people often do not realize just how stressful living with a serious, chronic ailment – such as thyroid disease – can prove. Yet some people live with very serious physical or mental illnesses, injury or trauma seemingly unscathed. Some even use adversity, illness and trauma as a springboard to personal growth. After all, adversity challenges your assumptions and forces you to examine your core beliefs. As such, adversity offers the opportunity and motivation to improve relationships, recognize new possibilities, increase appreciation for your blessings and aid spiritual development. My book *The Holistic Health Handbook* looks at these issues in depth.

In the *Handbook*, I look at the growing body of scientific studies indicating that hope, optimism and positive emotions generally may help restore your mental and physical resources, build long-lasting social resources and enhance well-being, despite intense stress. In addition, positive emotions increase your flexibility of thinking and enhance problem solving.[82] Remember that emotions are contagious. If you keep optimistic, it is more likely that the people around you will remain optimistic, creating a virtuous cycle.

Laughter is a medicine

Laughter helps create a constructive mental outlook that aids problem solving.[98] In addition, humour counters stress, depression, insomnia and loneliness, and enhances self-esteem, hope, mood, energy and vigour.[99,100] And laughter releases the tension generated by fear and anger, which are common reactions to living with thyroid disease. Likewise, tears discharge the tension that accompanies sadness linked to chronic disease. So curl up with a comedy DVD, CD or book. You may be able to have the last laugh over your thyroid disease.

Summing up

The American Psychological Association has proposed ten ways to help build resilience and help cope with the stress of living with a serious disease. (I slightly adapted these in *The Holistic Health Handbook* and have modified them further here to be more relevant to people with thyroid disease.) You can find the original at: <www.apa.org/helpcenter/road-resilience.aspx>.

Connections and relationships

Develop a network of supportive relationships with family, friends, voluntary and other groups, religious organizations and charities.

Many people find that helping others benefits them in times of difficulty and can distract them from the problems posed by living with thyroid disease or another chronic illness. Do not be afraid to express your emotions. Discuss your problems and accept help and support from other people.

You can overcome your problems

Your problems are not insurmountable. You cannot alter events in the past and if, for example, you have your thyroid gland removed or develop metastatic cancer, you may not be able to change the future. So try to accept your illness, your treatment or your problems. Even if you cannot change your circumstances nor do anything about your thyroid disease, you can alter how you react.

Accept that everything changes

The Greek philosopher Heraclitus famously commented about 2,500 years ago: 'Everything changes, nothing stays still ... You cannot step into the same stream twice.' You may need to accept that circumstances mean you may perhaps no longer be able to attain a once-treasured ambition. You may need to rethink your goals and re-evaluate your ambitions in the light of your thyroid-related symptoms or treatment.

On the other hand, there may be nothing you can do if, for example, you develop thyroid cancer or need surgery. So accept that some circumstances cannot be changed. Even for atheists, Reinhold Niebuhr's 'Serenity Prayer' eloquently sums up this approach: 'God, grant me the serenity to accept the things I cannot change / The courage to change the things I can / And the wisdom to know the difference.'

Develop and move towards realistic goals

Try to take small steps – every day if you can and even if it is a relatively small advance – that take you closer to your goal. Remember to break large goals into smaller steps and set a deadline. Counsellors can often help you define some new goals in light of your thyroid disease.

Do not be passive

Some people facing a problem, such as living with thyroid disease, withdraw excessively or hope their problems will sort themselves out. You need to identify your problems and take action. Being active helps engender a feeling that you are in control of your thyroid disease rather than your illness controlling you. You could explore complementary medicines, or new ways of drawing attention away from your thyroid eye disease or thinning hair, for example.

Make the most of the problem

A problem – even thyroid disease – can be part of your voyage of self-discovery. Many people experience 'post-traumatic growth' in their relationships, a sense of inner strength, self-worth, spirituality and a heightened appreciation for life.

Keep your problems in perspective

Try to take a broader view by, for example, focusing on other parts of your life rather than allowing your thyroid disease to dominate. Try to count your blessings – some people even make a list. Try not to make mountains out of molehills. You could ask yourself whether the problem will still be an issue in 6 months' or a year's time. Humour, literature and the other arts, visiting museums, walking in nature (page 118) can help create and maintain a sense of perspective.

Look after yourself

Ask yourself what you need to do to help yourself cope with the burden of living with thyroid disease. Find the time to take part in activities that you enjoy and to care for your appearance, which is especially useful if your thyroid disease is affecting the way you look. Try to exercise regularly, even if you feel tired – your energy levels should gradually improve. And make sure you get a good night's sleep (page 113). You may need to find the time to take a more active approach to relaxation (page 121).

Find other ways to bolster your inner resources

You could keep a diary, meditate or invest more time in your spiritual practices. Many people find that reading inspirational books from their or another religious tradition (even for atheists and agnostics), biographies, novels and so on helps them adapt to changes in their life. Don't underestimate the power of literature – or other arts – to educate, transform and inspire.

Stay positive

Develop confidence in your ability to solve problems arising from thyroid disease and your life in general, and trust your instincts. An active approach to tackling problems can help. Success breeds success. Moving towards your goal boosts your confidence and again helps you feel in control of your thyroid disease. Do not forget about the healing power of humour.

Nurture hope and optimism

Optimism and hope aid recovery. Try focusing on your goals rather than worrying about your anxieties or ruminating on your thyroid disease. But do not let this distract you from taking action to deal with your problems or finding the best way to live with your thyroid disease.

These may sound like platitudes, counsels of perfection and difficult to implement. But it's worth making the effort. Changing the way you cope with thyroid disease can transform your quality of life. After all, thyroid disease affects every part of your life: physical, mental and emotional. However, a combination of conventional treatments, lifestyle changes and complementary therapies can help you live an active and fulfilled life. I wish you well.

Useful addresses

Action on Smoking and Health (ASH)
Sixth Floor, Suites 59–63
New House, 67–68 Hatton Garden
London EC1N 8JY
Tel.: 020 7404 0242
Website: www.ash.org.uk

American Thyroid Association
Website: www.thyroid.org
While the site contains much valuable information, medical practice sometimes differs in the USA and UK.

British Association for Counselling and Psychotherapy (BACP)
BACP House
15 St John's Business Park
Lutterworth
Leics LE17 4HB
Tel.: 01455 883300
Website:www.bacp.co.uk

British Association of Endocrine and Thyroid Surgeons
C/o Association of Surgeons of Great Britain and Ireland
35–43 Lincoln's Inn Fields
London WC2A 3PE
Website: www.baets.org.uk

British Association of Medical Hypnosis
45 Hyde Park Square
London W2 2JT
Website: www.bamh.org.uk

British Dietetic Association
Fifth Floor, Charles House,
148/9 Great Charles Street
Queensway
Birmingham B3 3HT
Tel.: 0121 200 8080
Website: www.bda.uk.com

British Heart Foundation
Greater London House
180 Hampstead Road
London NW1 7AW
Tel.: 0300 330 3311 (helpline)
Website: www.bhf.org.uk

British Society of Gastroenterology
3 St Andrews Place
Regent's Park
London NW1 4LB
Tel.: 020 7935 3150
Website: www.bsg.org.uk

British Society for Paediatric Endocrinology and Diabetes
Contact via the website.
Website: www.bsped.org.uk

British Thyroid Association
Website:www.british-thyroid-association.org/
A learned society of professional clinical specialist doctors and scientists. It is not able to respond to individual medical questions and recommends that these should be directed to doctors, specialists or the British Thyroid Foundation (see below).

British Thyroid Foundation
Second Floor, 3 Devonshire Place
Harrogate
North Yorkshire HG1 4AA
Tel.: 01423 709707/709448
Website: www.btf-thyroid.org
A membership organization to help
people with thyroid disorders and
those supporting them.

Cancer Research UK
Angel Building
407 St John Street
London EC1V 4AD
Tel.: 0300 123 1022 (general
enquiries); 0808 800 4040
(helpline)
Website: www.cancerresearchuk.org

Macmillan Cancer Support
89 Albert Embankment
London SE1 7UQ
Tel.: 020 7840 7840 (general); 0808
808 00 00 (helpline)
Website: www.macmillan.org.uk

National Osteoporosis Society
Camerton
Bath BA2 0PJ
Tel.: 0845 130 3076 (general); 0845
450 0230 (helpline)
Website: www.nos.org.uk

**Royal National Institute of Blind
People**
105 Judd Street
London WC1H 9NE
Tel.: 0303 123 9999 (helpline)
Website: www.rnib.org.uk

**Thyroid Eye Disease Charitable
Trust**
PO Box 1928
Bristol BS37 0AX
Tel.: 0844 800 8133
Website: www.tedct.co.uk

Thyroid UK
32 Darcy Road
St Osyth
Clacton on Sea
Essex CO16 8QF
Tel.: 01255 820407 (10 a.m. to 2.30
p.m., Monday to Friday)
Website: www.thyroiduk.org.uk

References

1   Farling PA. Thyroid disease. *British Journal of Anaesthesia* 2000; **85**: 15–28.
2   Medeiros-Neto G, Camargo RY, Tomimori EK. Approach to and treatment of goiters. *Medical Clinics of North America* 2012; **96**: 351–68.
3   Leoutsakos V. A short history of the thyroid gland. *Hormones* 2004; **3**: 268–71.
4   Vanderpump MP, Tunbridge WMG. *Thyroid Disease: The Facts*. 4th ed. Oxford: Oxford University Press; 2008.
5   Taylor PN, Iqbal A, Minassian C, et al. Falling threshold for treatment of borderline elevated thyrotropin levels – balancing benefits and risks: evidence from a large community-based study. *JAMA Internal Medicine* 2014; **174**: 32–9.
6   Klein I, Danzi S. Thyroid disease and the heart. *Circulation* 2007; **116**: 1725–35.
7   Westcott P. *The Healthy Thyroid*. Revised ed. London: Thorsons; 2003.
8   Vanderpump MP. The epidemiology of thyroid disease. *British Medical Bulletin* 2011; **99**: 39–51.
9   Stagnaro-Green A, Sullivan S, Pearce EN. Iodine supplementation during pregnancy and lactation. *Journal of the American Medical Association* 2012; **308**: 2463–4.
10 Bath SC, Steer CD, Golding J, Emmett P, Rayman MP. Effect of inadequate iodine status in UK pregnant women on cognitive outcomes in their children: results from the Avon Longitudinal Study of Parents and Children (ALSPAC). *Lancet* 2013; **382**: 331–7.
11 Hynes KL, Otahal P, Hay I, Burgess JR. Mild iodine deficiency during pregnancy is associated with reduced educational outcomes in the offspring: 9-year follow-up of the Gestational Iodine Cohort. *Journal of Clinical Endocrinology and Metabolism* 2013; **98**: 1954–62.
12 Perlman R. *Evolution and Medicine*. Oxford: Oxford University Press; 2013.
13 Stojančević M, Bojić G, Salami HA, Mikov M. The influence of intestinal tract and probiotics on the fate of orally administered drugs. *Current Issues in Molecular Biology* 2013; **16**: 55–68.
14 Le Chatelier E, Nielsen T, Qin J, et al. Richness of human gut microbiome correlates with metabolic markers. *Nature* 2013; **500**: 541–6.
15 Zhu Q, Gao R, Wu W, Qin H. The role of gut microbiota in the pathogenesis of colorectal cancer. *Tumor Biology* 2013; **34**: 1285–300.
16 Dominguez LJ, Belvedere M, Barbagallo M. Thyroid Disorders. In: Sinclair AJ, Morley JE, Vellas B (eds), *Pathy's Principles and Practice of Geriatric Medicine*. Chichester: John Wiley & Sons; 2012, pp. 1183–97.
17 Stathatos N. Thyroid physiology. *Medical Clinics of North America* 2012; **96**: 165–73.
18 Brook CGD, Brown RS (eds). The thyroid gland. In: *Handbook of*

Clinical Pediatric Endocrinology. Oxford: Blackwell Publishing; 2008, pp. 84–98.

19 De Smet MP. Pathological anatomy of endemic goitre. *Monograph Series World Health Organization* 1960; **44**: 315–49.

20 Bianco MR, La Boria A, Franco T, Ferrise P, Allegra E. Ectopic lingual thyroid with vascular anomalies. *International Medical Case Reports Journal* 2013; **6**: 55–8.

21 Henderson J. Ernest Starling and 'Hormones': an historical commentary. *Journal of Endocrinology* 2005; **184**: 5–10.

22 Almandoz JP, Gharib H. Hypothyroidism: etiology, diagnosis, and management. *Medical Clinics of North America* 2012; **96**: 203–21.

23 Noiesen E, Trosborg I, Bager L, Herning M, Lyngby C, Konradsen H. Constipation – prevalence and incidence among medical patients acutely admitted to hospital with a medical condition. *Journal of Clinical Nursing* 2013 Dec 26 [Epub ahead of print].

24 Weetman A. Current choice of treatment for hypo- and hyperthyroidism. *Prescriber* 2013; **24**: 23–33.

25 Garg A, Vanderpump MP. Subclinical thyroid disease. *British Medical Bulletin* 2013; **107**: 101–16.

26 Gan EH, Pearce SH. Clinical review: the thyroid in mind: cognitive function and low thyrotropin in older people. *Journal of Clinical Endocrinology and Metabolism* 2012; **97**: 3438–49.

27 Budd M. *Why am I so Tired? Is your thyroid making you ill?* London: Thorsons; 2000.

28 Popoveniuc G, Jonklaas J. Thyroid nodules. *Medical Clinics of North America* 2012; **96**: 329–49.

29 Chatterjee VKK. Thyroid in 2012: advances in thyroid development, hormone action and neoplasia. *Nature Reviews Endocrinology* 2013; **9**: 74–6.

30 Leboulleux S, Borget I, Labro S, et al. Frequency and intensity of pain related to thyroid nodule fine-needle aspiration cytology. *Thyroid* 2013; **23**: 1113–18.

31 Castro MR. Multinodular goiter – diagnostic and treatment considerations. *US Endocrinology* 2008; 4. Available at: <www.touchendocrinology.com/articles/multinodular-goiter-diagnostic-and-treatment-considerations>.

32 Smith-Bindman R, Lebda P, Feldstein VA, et al. Risk of thyroid cancer based on thyroid ultrasound imaging characteristics: results of a population-based study. *JAMA Internal Medicine* 2013; **173**: 1788–96.

33 Annunziato A. DNA packaging: nucleosomes and chromatin. *Nature Education* 2008; **1**: 26. Available at: <www.nature.com/scitable/topicpage/dna-packaging-nucleosomes-and-chromatin-310>.

34 Hartl FU, Bracher A, Hayer-Hartl M. Molecular chaperones in protein folding and proteostasis. *Nature* 2011; **475**: 324–32.

35 Duclos A, Peix J-L, Colin C, et al. Influence of experience on performance of individual surgeons in thyroid surgery: prospective cross sectional multicentre study. *British Medical Journal* 2012; **344**: d8041.

36 Pedullá M, Fierro V, Papacciuolo V, Alfano R, Ruocco E. Atopy as a risk factor for thyroid autoimmunity in children affected with atopic dermatitis. *Journal of the European Academy of Dermatology and Venereology* 2013 Oct 3 [Epub ahead of print].

37 Hunt RH, Dhaliwal S, Tougas G, et al. Prevalence, impact and attitudes toward lower gastrointestinal dysmotility and sensory symptoms, and their treatment in Canada: a descriptive study. *Canadian Journal of Gastroenterology* 2007; **21**: 31–7.

38 Malagelada JR. A symptom-based approach to making a positive diagnosis of irritable bowel syndrome with constipation. *International Journal of Clinical Practice* 2006; **60**: 57–63.

39 Stuijver DJF, Piantanida E, van Zaane B, et al. Acquired von Willebrand syndrome in patients with overt hypothyroidism: a prospective cohort study. *Haemophilia* 2014; **20**: 326–32.

40 Falgarone G, Heshmati HM, Cohen R, Reach G. Mechanisms in endocrinology. Role of emotional stress in the pathophysiology of Graves' disease. *European Journal of Endocrinology* 2013; **168**: R13–18.

41 Lazarus JH. Thyroid function in pregnancy. *British Medical Bulletin* 2011; **97**: 137–48.

42 Hemminki K, Li X, Sundquist J, Sundquist K. The epidemiology of Graves' disease: evidence of a genetic and an environmental contribution. *Journal of Autoimmunity* 2010; **34**: J307–13.

43 Benjamin EJ, Chen PS, Bild DE, et al. Prevention of atrial fibrillation: report from a National Heart, Lung, and Blood Institute workshop. *Circulation* 2009; **119**: 606–18.

44 Mulder BJ, van der Wall EE. Size and function of the atria. *International Journal of Cardiovascular Imaging* 2008; **24**: 713–16.

45 Azoulay L, Dell'Aniello S, Simon TA, Renoux C, Suissa S. Initiation of warfarin in patients with atrial fibrillation: early effects on ischaemic strokes. *European Heart Journal* 2013 Dec 18 [Epub ahead of print].

46 Tjiang H, Lahooti H, McCorquodale T, Parmar KR, Wall JR. Eye and eyelid abnormalities are common in patients with Hashimoto's thyroiditis. *Thyroid* 2010; **20**: 287–90.

47 Perros P, Crombie AL, Kendall-Taylor P. Natural history of thyroid associated ophthalmopathy. *Clinical Endocrinology* 1995; **42**: 45–50.

48 Hajdu SI. A note from history: landmarks in history of cancer, part 3. *Cancer* 2012; **118**: 1155–68.

49 Parkin DM. 2. Tobacco-attributable cancer burden in the UK in 2010. *British Journal of Cancer* 2011; **105**: S6–13.

50 Vestergaard P, Rejnmark L, Weeke J, et al. Smoking as a risk factor for Graves' disease, toxic nodular goiter, and autoimmune hypothyroidism. *Thyroid* 2002; **12**: 69–75.

51 Montgomery GH, Schnur JB, Kravits K. Hypnosis for cancer care: over 200 years young. *CA: A Cancer Journal for Clinicians* 2013; **63**: 31–44.

52 Aubin H-J, Farley A, Lycett D, Lahmek P, Aveyard P. Weight gain in smokers after quitting cigarettes: meta-analysis. *British Medical Journal* 2012; **345**: e4439.

53 Marcocci C, Kahaly GJ, Krassas GE, et al. Selenium and the course of

mild Graves' orbitopathy. *New England Journal of Medicine* 2011; **364**: 1920–31.

54 Pacini F, Castagna MG, Brilli L, Pentheroudakis G. Thyroid cancer: ESMO Clinical Practice Guidelines for diagnosis, treatment and follow-up. *Annals of Oncology* 2012; **23** Suppl 7: vii 10–19.

55 Brown T, Young C, Rushton L. Occupational cancer in Britain. Remaining cancer sites: brain, bone, soft tissue sarcoma and thyroid. *British Journal of Cancer* 2012; **107** Suppl 1: S85–91.

56 dos Santos Silva I, Swerdlow AJ. Thyroid cancer epidemiology in England and Wales: time trends and geographical distribution. *British Journal of Cancer* 1993; **67**: 330–40.

57 Luo J, Sands M, Wactawski-Wende J, Song Y, Margolis KL. Sleep disturbance and incidence of thyroid cancer in postmenopausal women. The Women's Health Initiative. *American Journal of Epidemiology* 2013; **177**: 42–9.

58 Han JM, Kim TY, Jeon MJ, et al. Obesity is a risk factor for thyroid cancer in a large, ultrasonographically screened population. *European Journal of Endocrinology* 2013; **168**: 879–86.

59 Reiners C, Biko J, Haenscheid H, et al. Twenty-five years after Chernobyl: outcome of radioiodine treatment in children and adolescents with very-high-risk radiation-induced differentiated thyroid carcinoma. *Journal of Clinical Endocrinology and Metabolism* 2013; **98**: 3039–48.

60 van den Boogaard E, Vissenberg R, Land JA, et al. Significance of (sub)clinical thyroid dysfunction and thyroid autoimmunity before conception and in early pregnancy: a systematic review. *Human Reproduction Update* 2011; **17**: 605–19.

61 Vissenberg R, van den Boogaard E, van Wely M, et al. Treatment of thyroid disorders before conception and in early pregnancy: a systematic review. *Human Reproduction Update* 2012; **18**: 360–73.

62 Román GC, Ghassabian A, Bongers-Schokking JJ, et al. Association of gestational maternal hypothyroxinemia and increased autism risk. *Annals of Neurology* 2013; **74**: 733–42.

63 Su VY-F, Hu Y-W, Chou K-T, et al. Amiodarone and the risk of cancer. *Cancer* 2013; **119**: 1699–705.

64 Whybrow PC, Bauer M. Depression, mania, and thyroid function: a story of intimate relationships. In: Licinio J, Wong M-L (eds), *Biology of Depression*. Weinheim, Germany: Wiley-VCH; 2008, pp. 523–37.

65 Iglesias P, Ridruejo E, Muñoz A, et al. Thyroid function tests and mortality in aged hospitalized patients: a 7-year prospective observational study. *Journal of Clinical Endocrinology and Metabolism* 2013; **98**: 4683–9.

66 Tran HA. The swinging thyroid in hepatitis C infection and interferon therapy. *QJM* 2010; **103**: 187–91.

67 Mouritsen O. The science of seaweeds. *American Scientist* 2013; **101**: 458–63.

68 Yokoyama M, Origasa H, Matsuzaki M, et al. Effects of eicosapentaenoic acid on major coronary events in hypercholesterolaemic patients

(JELIS): a randomised open-label, blinded endpoint analysis. *Lancet* 2007; **369**: 1090–8.

69 Malhotra A. Saturated fat is not the major issue. *British Medical Journal* 2013; **347**: f6340.

70 Abramson JD, Rosenberg HG, Jewell N, et al. Should people at low risk of cardiovascular disease take a statin? *BMJ* 2013; **347**: f6123.

71 Ito MK, Maki KC, Brinton EA, Cohen JD, Jacobson TA. Muscle symptoms in statin users, associations with cytochrome P450, and membrane transporter inhibitor use: a subanalysis of the USAGE study. *Journal of Clinical Lipidology* 2014; **8**: 69–76.

72 De Giorgio R, Barbara G, Stanghellini V, et al. Diagnosis and therapy of irritable bowel syndrome. *Alimentary Pharmacology and Therapeutics* 2004; **20**: 10–22.

73 National Institute for Health and Care Excellence. *Irritable bowel syndrome in adults: diagnosis and management of irritable bowel syndrome in primary care.* NICE clinical guideline 61. February 2008. Available at: <http://guidance.nice.org.uk/CG61/NICEGuidance/pdf/English>.

74 Lopez-Munoz F, Alamo C. Monoaminergic neurotransmission: the history of the discovery of antidepressants from 1950s until today. *Current Pharmaceutical Design* 2009; **15**: 1563–86.

75 Rush AJ, Trivedi MH, Wisniewski SR, et al. Acute and longer-term outcomes in depressed outpatients requiring one or several treatment steps: a STAR*D report. *American Journal of Psychiatry* 2006; **163**: 1905–17.

76 Lam RW. Sleep disturbances and depression: a challenge for antidepressants. *International Clinical Psychopharmacology* 2006; **21** Suppl 1: S25–9.

77 Bower B. DSM-5 enters the diagnostic fray. *Science News* 2013; **183**: 5–6.

78 Dowben JS, Grant JS, Keltner NL. Ketamine as an alternative treatment for treatment-resistant depression. *Perspectives in Psychiatric Care* 2013; **49**: 2–4.

79 Buffoli B, Rinaldi F, Labanca M, et al. The human hair: from anatomy to physiology. *International Journal of Dermatology* 2014; **53**: 331–41.

80 Waite LJ, Lehrer EL. The benefits from marriage and religion in the United States: a comparative analysis. *Population and Development Review* 2003; **29**: 255–76.

81 Siegler IC, Brummett BH, Martin P, Helms MJ. Consistency and timing of marital transitions and survival during midlife: the role of personality and health risk behaviors. *Annals of Behavioral Medicine* 2013; **45**: 338–47.

82 Ong AD, Bergeman CS, Boker SM. Resilience comes of age: defining features in later adulthood. *Journal of Personality* 2009; **77**: 1777–804.

83 Kravdal H, Syse A. Changes over time in the effect of marital status on cancer survival. *BMC Public Health* 2011; **11**: 804.

84 Franks MM, Stephens MA, Rook KS, Franklin BA, Keteyian SJ, Artinian NT. Spouses' provision of health-related support and control to

patients participating in cardiac rehabilitation. *Journal of Family Psychology* 2006; **20**: 311–18.

85 Kiecolt-Glaser JK, Loving TJ, Stowell JR, et al. Hostile marital interactions, proinflammatory cytokine production, and wound healing. *Archives of General Psychiatry* 2005; **62**: 1377–84.

86 Vallance AK. Something out of nothing: the placebo effect. *Advances in Psychiatric Treatment* 2006; **12**: 287–96.

87 Tsunetsugu Y, Park B-J, Miyazaki Y. Trends in research related to 'Shinrin-yoku' (taking in the forest atmosphere or forest bathing) in Japan. *Environmental Health and Preventive Medicine* 2010; **15**: 27–37.

88 Restriction of hypnotic performances. *British Medical Journal* 1890; **1**: 1264.

89 Singh P, Singh B, Dave R, Udainiya R. The impact of yoga upon female patients suffering from hypothyroidism. *Complementary Therapies in Clinical Practice* 2011; **17**: 132–4.

90 Swami G, Singh S, Singh KP, Gupta M. Effect of yoga on pulmonary function tests of hypothyroid patients. *Indian Journal of Physiology and Pharmacology* 2010; **54**: 51–6.

91 Donesky-Cuenco D, Nguyen HQ, Paul S, Carrieri-Kohlman V. Yoga therapy decreases dyspnea-related distress and improves functional performance in people with chronic obstructive pulmonary disease: a pilot study. *Journal of Alternative and Complementary Medicine* 2009; **15**: 225–34.

92 Cramer H, Lauche R, Hohmann C, Langhorst J, Dobos G. Yoga for chronic neck pain: a 12-month follow-up. *Pain Med* 2013; **14**: 541–8.

93 Streeter CC, Whitfield TH, Owen L, et al. Effects of yoga versus walking on mood, anxiety, and brain GABA levels: a randomized controlled MRS study. *Journal of Alternative and Complementary Medicine* 2010; **16**: 1145–52.

94 Goes TC, Antunes FD, Alves PB, Teixeira-Silva F. Effect of sweet orange aroma on experimental anxiety in humans. *Journal of Alternative and Complementary Medicine* 2012; **18**: 798–804.

95 Sveinsdottir V, Eriksen HR, Reme SE. Assessing the role of cognitive behavioral therapy in the management of chronic nonspecific back pain. *Journal of Pain Research* 2012; **5**: 371–80.

96 Singh A. Use of mindfulness-based therapies in psychiatry. *Progress in Neurology and Psychiatry* 2012; **16**: 7–11.

97 Wiles N, Thomas L, Abel A, et al. Cognitive behavioural therapy as an adjunct to pharmacotherapy for primary care based patients with treatment resistant depression: results of the CoBalT randomised controlled trial. *Lancet* 2012; **381**: 375–84.

98 Dugan DO. Laughter and tears: best medicine for stress. *Nursing Forum* 1989; **24**: 18–26.

99 Takeda M, Hashimoto R, Kudo T, et al. Laughter and humor as complementary and alternative medicines for dementia patients. *BMC Complementary and Alternative Medicine* 2010; **10**: 28.

100 Mora-Ripoll R. The therapeutic value of laughter in medicine. *Alternative Therapies in Health and Medicine* 2010; **16**: 56–64.

Further reading

Roberta Bivins. *Alternative Medicine? A history*. Oxford: Oxford University Press; 2007.

Bill Bryson. *A Short History of Nearly Everything*. London: Black Swan; 2003.

Martin Budd. *Why am I so Tired? Is your thyroid making you ill?* London: Thorsons; 2000.

Mark Greener. *Coping with Liver Disease*. London: Sheldon Press; 2013.

Mark Greener. *The Heart Attack Survival Guide*. London: Sheldon Press; 2011.

Mark Greener. *The Holistic Health Handbook*. London: Sheldon Press; 2013.

Mark Greener and Christine Craggs-Hinton. *The Diabetes Healing Diet*. London: Sheldon Press; 2012.

Anne Harrington. *The Cure Within: A history of mind–body medicine*. New York: W. W. Norton; 2008.

Stephen E. Langer and James F. Scheer. *Solved: The Riddle of Illness*. 2nd ed. New Canaan, CT, USA: Keats; 1995.

Mary Roach. *Gulp: Adventures on the Alimentary Canal*. London: Oneworld; 2013.

Andrew Russell. *The Social Basis of Medicine*. Chichester: Wiley Blackwell; 2009.

Mark Vanderpump and Michael Tunbridge. *Thyroid Disease: The Facts*. 4th ed. Oxford: Oxford University Press; 2008.

Patsy Westcott. *The Healthy Thyroid*. Revised ed. London: Thorsons; 2003.

Index